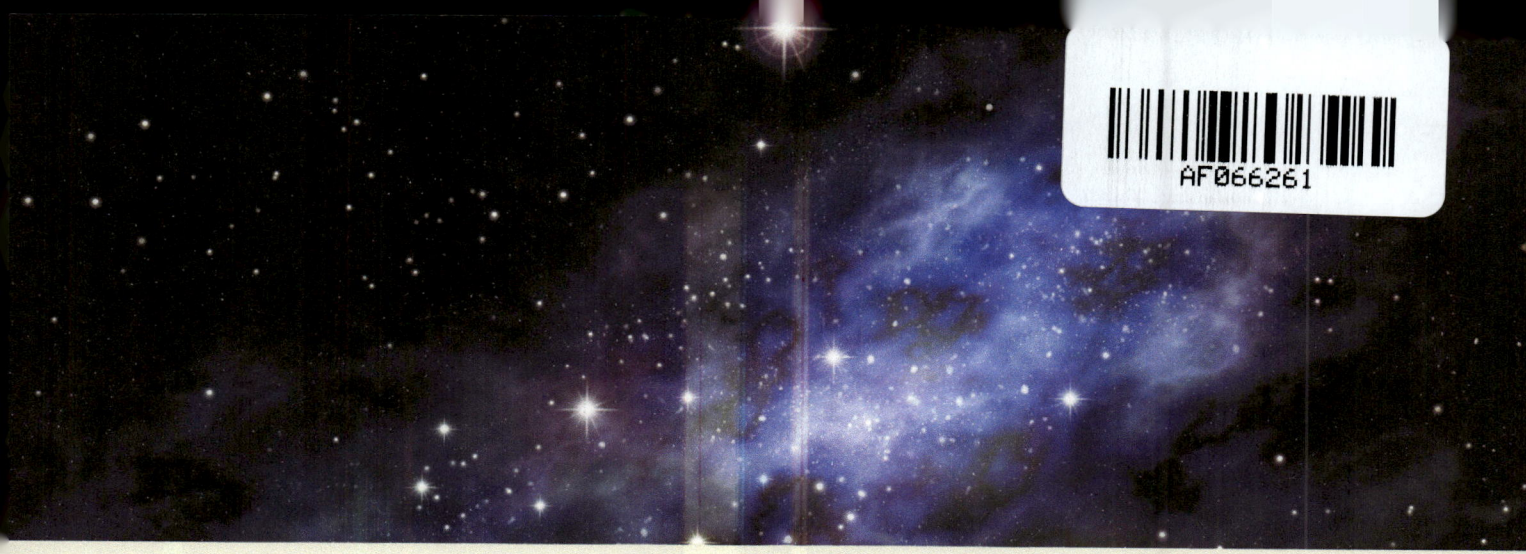

Push your Career Publish your Thesis

Science should be accessible to everybody. Share the knowledge, the ideas, and the passion about your research. Give your part of the infinite amount of scientific research possibilities a finite frame.

Publish your examination paper, diploma thesis, bachelor thesis, master thesis, dissertation, or habilitation treatises in form of a book.

A finite frame by infinite science.

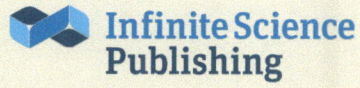

An Imprint of
Infinite Science GmbH
MFC 1 | Technikzentrum Lübeck
BioMedTec Wissenschaftscampus
Maria-Goeppert-Straße 1
23562 Lübeck
book@infinite-science.de
www.infinite-science.de

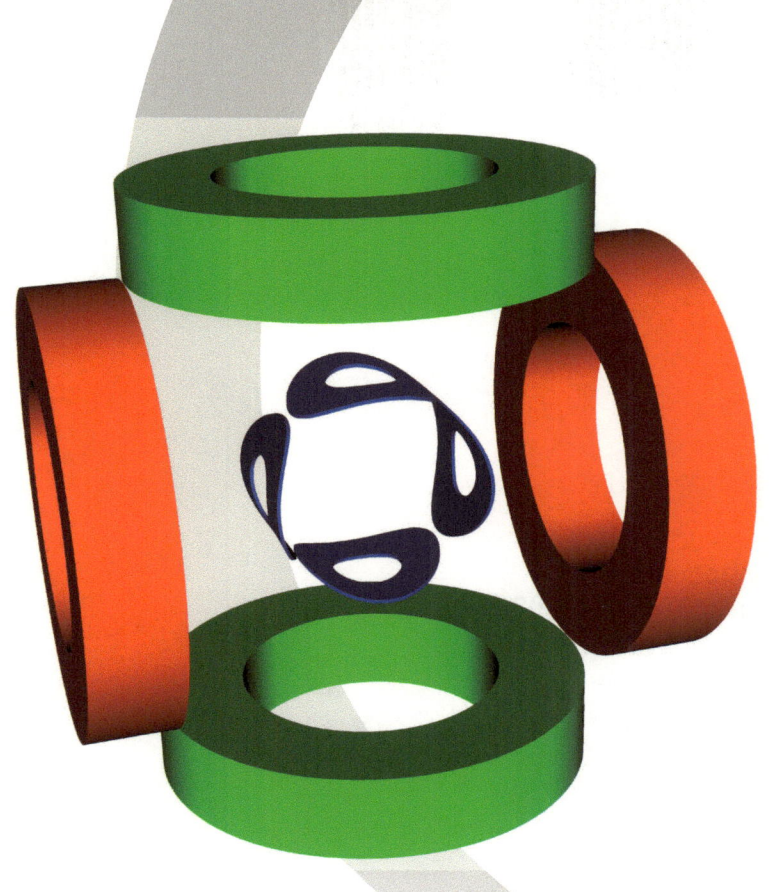

4th International Workshop on
Magnetic Particle Imaging
IWMPI 2014

March 27 - 29, 2014

Berlin, Germany

BOOK OF ABSTRACTS

T. M. Buzug, J. Borgert (Eds.)

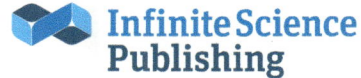

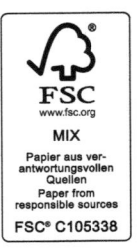

International Workshop on Magnetic Particle Imaging (IWMPI2014) Book of Abstracts (2nd Edition)

Editors:
Thorsten M. Buzug, Jörn Borgert

© 2015 Infinite Science Publishing
der BioMedTec Wissenschaftsverlag Lübeck

An Imprint of Infinite Science GmbH,
MFC 1 | BioMedTec Wissenschaftscampus
Maria-Goeppert-Straße 1
23562 Lübeck

Umschlaggestaltung, Illustration: Uli Schmidts, metonym
Lektorat: Universität zu Lübeck, Institut für Medizintechnik

Verlag: Infinite Science GmbH, Lübeck, www.infinite-science.de
Druck: Books on Demand GmbH, Norderstedt

ISBN Paperback 978-3-945954-01-0   -   2. Auflage

Das Werk, einschließlich seiner Teile, ist urheberrechtlich geschützt. Jede Verwertung ist ohne Zustimmung des Verlages und des Autors unzulässig. Dies gilt insbesondere für die elektronische oder sonstige Vervielfältigung, Bearbeitung, Übersetzung, Mikroverfilmung, Verbreitung und öffentliche Zugänglichmachung sowie die Einspeicherung und Verarbeitung in elektronischen Systemen.

Die Wiedergabe von Gebrauchsnamen, Handelsnamen, Warenbezeichnungen usw. in dieser Publikation berechtigt auch ohne besondere Kennzeichnung nicht zu der Annahme, dass solche Namen im Sinne der Warenzeichen- und Markenschutz-Gesetzgebung als frei zu betrachten wären und daher von jedermann verwendet werden dürften.

Bibliografische Information der Deutschen Nationalbibliothek:
Die Deutsche Nationalbibliothek verzeichnet diese Publikation in der Deutschen Nationalbibliografie; detaillierte bibliografische Daten sind im Internet über http://dnb.d-nb.de abrufbar.

Bibliographic information published by the Deutsche Nationalbibliothek
The Deutsche Nationalbibliothek lists this publication in the Deutsche Nationalbibliografie; detailed bibliographic data are available in the internet at http://dnb.d-nb.de.

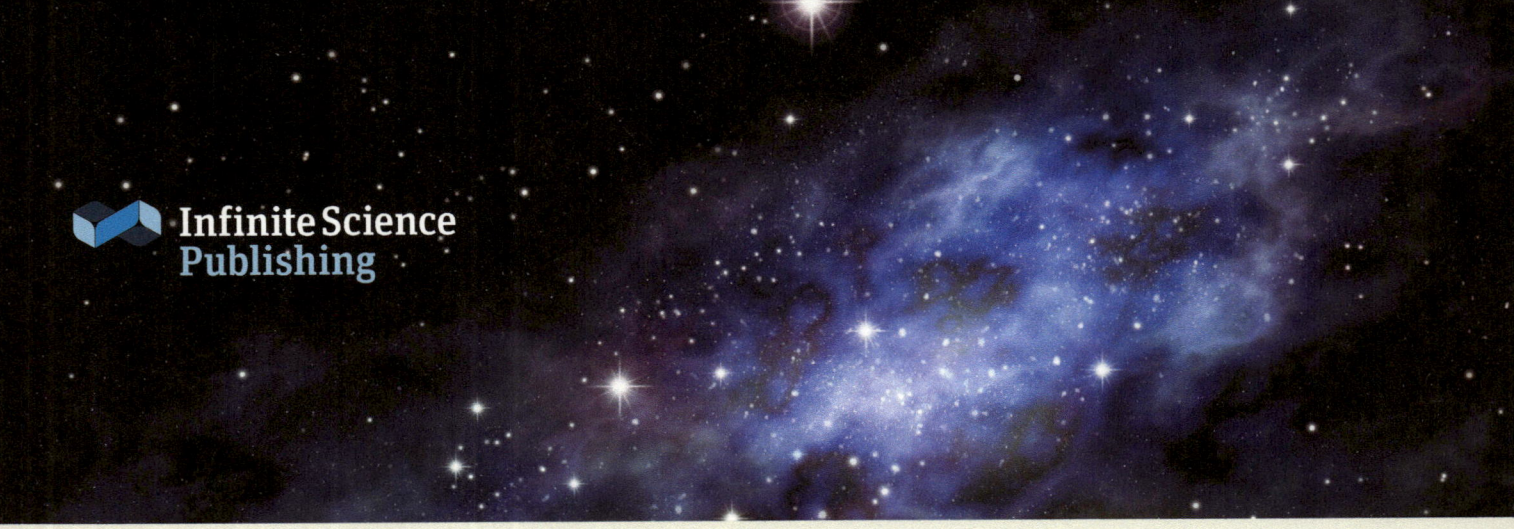

Wir verlegen Ihre wissenschaftlichen Schriften

Bachelor- und Masterarbeiten,
Dissertationen und Habilitationen,
Monografien und Tagungsbände, etc.

Kostenlose Verlegung als Buch mit ISBN-Nummer und Aufnahme in die Deutsche Nationalbibliothek

Hochwertiger Buchdruck in nachhaltiger Produktion (FSC-zertifiziert)

Günstiger Bezug von Autorenexemplaren
Weltweite Präsenz Ihres Werkes bei den großen Händlern: Amazon, Thalia, Hugendubel, Barnes & Noble u.v.m. sowie optional als eBook

www.infinite-science.de/publishing

Infinite Science GmbH
MFC 1 | BioMedTec Wissenschaftscampus
Maria-Goeppert-Str. 1, 23562 Lübeck
book@infinite-science.de

Locations and Travel Information

IWMPI 2014 will take place at two different locations, „Physikalisch-Technische Bundesanstalt" (PTB) Berlin Charlottenburg (March 27, 2014) and Charité Campus Virchow Klinikum (March 28 -29, 2014).

Local organization committee:
In urgent cases you can call us on +49 160 467 8174.

Thursday, March 27, 2014

Physikalisch-Technische Bundesanstalt (PTB) Berlin-Charlottenburg

Registration, Tutorials, Welcome Reception

Address:
Hermann-von-Helmholtz-Bau
Abbestraße 1
10587 Berlin

Friday, March 28, 2014

Charité Campus Virchow Klinikum (CVK)

Talks and Poster Sessions

Address:
see Saturday

Wasserwerk

Evening Event and Poster Award

Address:
Hohenzollerndamm 208,
10713 Berlin

Saturday, March 29, 2014

Charité Campus Virchow Klinikum (CVK)

Talks and Poster Sessions, Closing Remarks

Campus address:
Charité Campus Virchow-Klinikum
Augustenburger Platz 1
13353 Berlin

Internal address:
CVK, Forum 3

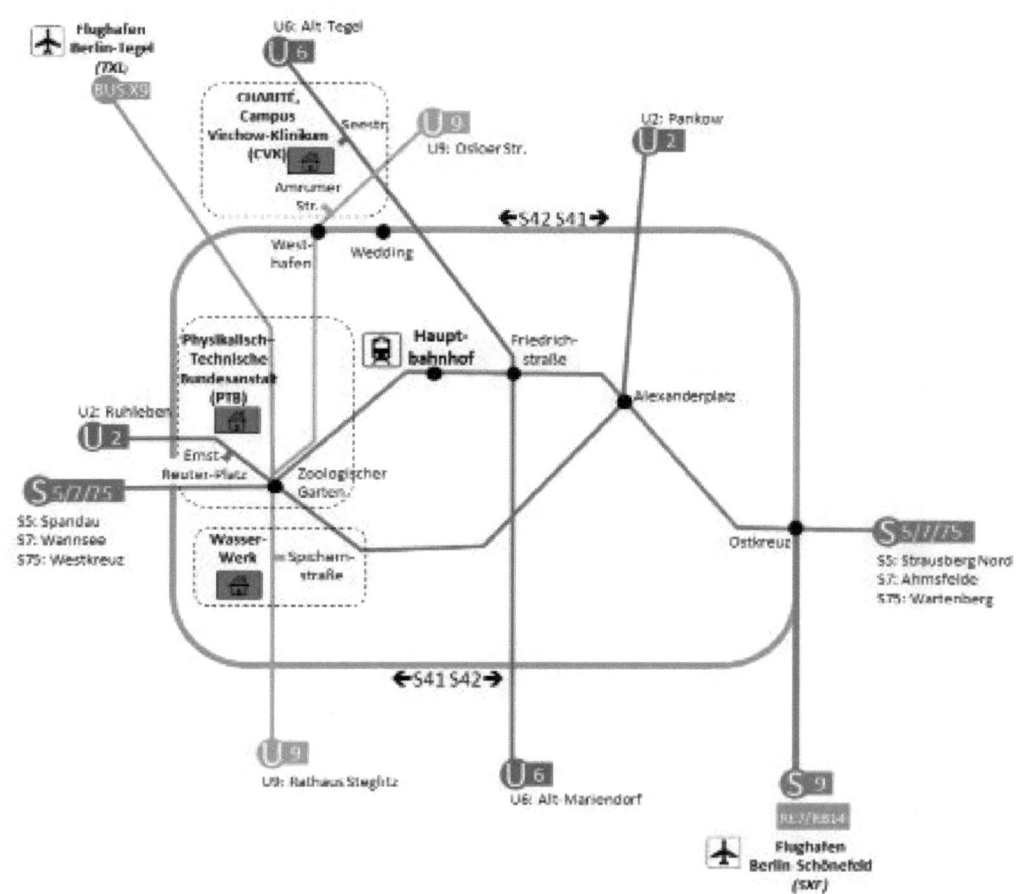

Scientific Program

Thursday, March 27, 2014 — Physikalisch-Technische Bundesanstalt (PTB)

14:00 - 18:00	Registration, Upload Presentations	

14:30 - 18:00 Tutorials

14:30 - 16:00	Tutorial 1: **Introduction to MPI**
	Field Design and Instrumentation
	Image Reconstruction Process
16:00 - 16:30	Coffee Break
16:30 - 18:00	Tutorial 2: **Magnetic Tracer Materials**
	Chemical, Biochemical, and Physiological Aspects
	Physics of Magnetic Tracer Materials

18:30 - 22:00 Welcome Reception with Live Music

Friday, March 28, 2014 — Charité Campus Virchow-Klinikum

08:00 - 09:00	Registration, Setup of Poster Presentation and Industry Exhibition

09:00 - 09:15	**Welcome Note**
	Thorsten M. Buzug; University of Lübeck
	Jörn Borgert; Philips Research Europe, Hamburg

09:15 - 09:45	**Opening Note**
	Prof. Karl M. Einhäupl; Charité - Universitätsmedizin Berlin

09:45 - 11:15	**Magnetic Particle Imaging I**
	Chairs: V. Behr, F. Ludwig
09:45 - 10:15	Challenges in the Application of Magnetic Particle Imaging
	Keynote Speech: Bernhard Gleich
10:15 - 10:30	Integrated TWMPI-MRI Hybrid Scanner
	P. Klauer; Experimental Physics 5 (Biophysics), University of Würzburg
10:30 - 10:45	Spin Electronics Based Sensors for Low Frequency Magnetic Signal Detection
	C. Fermon; CEA Saclay
10:45 - 11:00	Drive-Field Decoupling and Control Network for Magnetic Particle Imaging
	J. Franke; Bruker BioSpin MRI GmbH
11:00 - 11:15	X-Space Image Reconstruction Algorithm with Optimized 2D/3D DC Recovery
	J. Konkle; University of California, Berkeley

11:15 - 12:15	**Poster Session I (List of Posters see Page XVIII)**

| 12:15 - 13:00 | Lunch Break | |

13:00 - 14:15	**Imaging Technology and Safety** Chairs: O. Dössel, S. Conolly	
13:00 - 13:15	Imaging of MNP Using a Second Harmonic of Magnetization with DC Bias Field S. Tanaka; Toyohashi University of Technology	
13:15 - 13:30	Water-Cooled Two-Axis Rigid Excitation Coil Assembly P. Goodwill; University of California, Berkeley	
13:30 - 13:45	Considerations on Safety Limits for Magnetic Fields Used in Magnetic Particle Imaging O. Doessel; University of Karlsruhe	
13:45 - 14:00	MPI Safety in the View of MRI Safety Norms I. Schmale; Philips Technology GmbH, Hamburg	
14:00 - 14:15	Strategies for Fast MPI within the Limits Determined by Nerve Stimulation J. Rahmer; Philips Technology GmbH, Hamburg	

| 14:15 - 15:00 | Coffee Break | |

15:00 - 16:30	**Modelling, Simulation, Reconstruction & Sequences** Chairs: J. Weizenecker, B. Gleich	
15:00 - 15:30	UC Berkeley Innovations in MPI Hardware, Image Reconstruction; and Nanoparticles, with Application to Quantitative In Vivo Stem Cell Tracking **Keynote Speech: Steven Conolly**	
15:30 - 15:45	Compressed Sensing and Sparse Reconstruction in MPI A. von Gladiß; Institute of Medical Engineering, University of Lübeck	
15:45 - 16:00	Reconstruction Enhancement By Using Frequency Domain Filters A. Weber; Bruker BioSpin MRI	
16:00 - 16:15	A Phenomenological Description of the MPS-Signal Using a Model for the Field Dependence of the Effective Relaxation Time D. Schmidt; Physikalisch-Technische Bundesanstalt	
16:15 - 16:30	Debye-Based Frequency-Domain Magnetization Model for Magnetic Nanoparticles and its Application to Viscosity-Dependent MPS Measurements T. Wawrzik; TU Braunschweig	

| 16:30 - 17:00 | Coffee Break | |

17:00 - 18:00	**MPI Theory, Relaxometry, Magnetometry** Chairs: J. Weaver, L. Trahms	
17:00 - 17:15	Simultaneous Reconstruction and Resolution Enhancement for Magnetic Particle Imaging O. Omer; Institute of Medical Engineering, University of Lübeck	
17:15 - 17:30	Field Dependent Characteristic Timescales for Magnetic Nanoparticle Rotations D. Reeves; Dartmouth College	
17:30 - 17:45	Dependence of Brownian and Néel Relaxation Times on Magnetic Field Strength R. Deissler; Case Western Reserve University	
17:45 - 18:00	Handheld Differential Magnetometry with a Split Coil Geometry S. Waanders; MIRA Institute for Biomedical Technology and Technical Medicine	

| 19:00 - 01:00 | **Evening Event, Poster Award (Event Location Wasserwerk)** | |

Saturday, March 29, 2014 — Charité Campus Virchow-Klinikum

09:00 - 10:30	**Magnetic Nanoparticles & Tracer Materials** Chairs: G. Schuetz, M. Taupitz
09:00 - 09:30	Optimized tracers for MPI: Progress and Challenges **Keynote Speech: Kannan Krishnan**
09:30 - 09:45	Dynamic Magnetic Behaviour of DDM128 in Agarose Gel, Gelatine and Sugar Matrix *D. Eberbeck; Physikalisch-Technische Bundesanstalt*
09:45 - 10:00	Dependence of Temperature Probing on Taylor's Expansion of Langevin Function Using Magnetic Nanoparticles in DC Field *Ling Jiang; Huazhong University of Science and Technology*
10:00 - 10:15	Synthetic Approaches for Iron Oxide Nanoparticles Suitable as Tracer for Magnetic Particle Imaging *A. Ide; Bayer HealthCare Pharmaceuticals*
10:15 - 10:30	Perpendicular Magnetic Particle Imaging, pMPI *J. Weaver; Dartmouth College and Dartmouth-Hitchcock Medical Center*

10:30 - 11:15	Coffee Break

11:15 - 12:30	**Magnetic Nanoparticles & Tracer Materials** Chairs: K. Krishnan, J. Niehaus
11:15 - 11:30	Optimized MPI Tracers Perform Well Over a Range of Excitation Field Conditions *M. Ferguson; LodeSpin labs*
11:30 - 11:45	Hydrodynamic Fractionation to Enhance MPI Performance of Resovist® *N. Löwa; Physikalisch-Technische Bundesanstalt*
11:45 - 12:00	Magnetic Characterisation of Clustered Core Magnetic Nanoparticles for MPI *D. Heinke; nanoPET Pharma GmbH*
12:00 - 12:15	Tuning Magnetic Dipolar Interaction for Enhancing Magnetic Particle Imaging Performance *S. Sarangi; St. John's Research Institute, Bangalore*
12:15 - 12:30	Tuning Surface Coatings of Optimized Magnetite Nanoparticle Tracers for *In Vivo* MPI *A. Khandhar; University of Washington*

12:30 - 13:15	Lunch Break

13:15 - 14:15	**Poster Session II (List of Posters see Page XVIII)**

14:15 - 15:45		**Medical Applications** Chairs: M. Magnani, J. Barkhausen
14:15 - 14:45		Challenges for MPI: What are the Requirements a New Diagnostic Tool Must Meet? **Keynote Speech: Matthias Taupitz**
14:45 - 15:00		Stem Cell Vitality Assessment Using Magnetic Particle Spectroscopy *F. Fidler; Research Center Magnetic-Resonance-Bavaria*
15:00 - 15:15		Magnetic Particle Imaging (MPI): Visualization and Quantification of Vascular Stenosis Phantoms *J. Hägele; Clinic for Radiology and Nuclear Medicine, University Hospital Schleswig Holstein*
15:15 - 15:30		Time-Evolution Contrast of Target MRI Using Antibody Functionalized Magnetic Nanoparticles: An Animal Model *S. Yang; MagQu Co., Ltd.*
15:30 - 15:45		*In Vivo* MPI Neural Cell Monitoring in the Rat Brain *B. Zheng; University of California, Berkeley*

15:45 - 16:30	Coffee Break

16:30 - 17:30	**Magnetic Particle Imaging II** Chairs: U. Heinen, D. Baumgarten
16:30 - 16:45	Flow Assessment from *In Vitro* and *In Silico* Dynamic MPI Data *R. Lacroix; Philips Research Paris*
16:45 - 17:00	Two Dimensional Magnetic Particle Imaging With a Dynamic Field Free Line Scanner *K. Bente;Institute of Medical Engineering, University of Lübeck*
17:00 - 17:15	Concept of a Generator for the Selection- and Focus Field of a Clinical MPI Scanner *C. Bontus; Philips Technologie GmbH, Innovative Technologies, Research Laboratories*
17:15 - 17:30	Ultra High Resolution MPI *P. Vogel; Experimental Physics 5 (Biophysics), University of Würzburg*

17:30 - 17:45	**Closing Remarks** Thorsten M. Buzug; University of Lübeck Jörn Borgert; Philips Research Europe, Hamburg

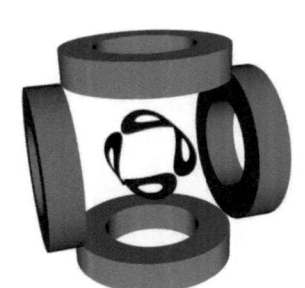

4th International Workshop on
Magnetic Particle Imaging
IWMPI 2014
March 27 - 29, 2014

Berlin, Germany

BOOK OF ABSTRACTS

Commitees

Workshop Chairs
Thorsten M. Buzug, Universität zu Lübeck
Jörn Borgert, Philips Research Europe - Hamburg

Local Chairs
Matthias Taupitz, Charité Berlin
Lutz Trahms, PTB Berlin

Organization
Kanina Botterweck, Medisert GmbH, Lübeck
Helmut Kunze, HealthCapital Berlin Brandenburg

Program Committee

G. Adam, UKE Hamburg
C. Alexiou, University of Erlangen
J. Barkhausen, UKSH Lübeck
V. Behr, University of Würzburg
J. Borgert, Philips Research Europe, Hamburg
J. Bulte, John Hopkins University, Baltimore
T. M. Buzug, University of Lübeck
S. M. Conolly, University of California, Berkeley
O. Dössel, University of Karlsruhe
S. Dutz, IPHT Jena
M. Ferguson, University of Washington
D. Finas, EVKB Bielefeld
B. Gleich, Philips Technology GmbH, Hamburg
P. W. Goodwill, University of California, Berkeley
M. Griswold, Case Western Reserve University, Cleveland
U. Häfeli, University of British Columbia, Vancouver
J. Haueisen, Ilmenau University of Technology
M. Heidenreich, Bruker BioSpin, Ettlingen
U. Heinen, Bruker BioSpin, Ettlingen
Y. Ishihara, Meiji University
P. Jakob, University of Würzburg
F. Kießling, University of Aachen
T. Knopp, Thorlabs, Lübeck
K. Krishnan, University of Washington
F. Ludwig, TU Braunschweig
M. Magnani, University of Urbino
S. Odenbach, TU Dresden
Q. Pankhurst, Davy-Faraday Research Laboratory, London
U. Pison, Charité Berlin
J. Rahmer, Philips Technology GmbH, Hamburg
A. Samia, Case Western Reserve University, Cleveland
E. U. Saritas, University of California, Berkeley
M. Schilling, Braunschweig University of Technology
I. Schmale, Philips Technology GmbH, Hamburg
J. Schnorr, Charité Berlin
G. Schuetz, Bayer HealthCare, Berlin
M. Taupitz, Charité Berlin
B. ten Haken, University of Twente
L. Trahms, PTB Berlin
J. Weaver, Dartmouth-Hitchcock Medical Center, Lebanon
J. Weizenecker, Karlsruhe University of Applied Sciences
H. Weller, CAN Hamburg
F. Wiekhorst, PTB Berlin

Preface and Acknowledgements

Dear colleagues,

after the great success of IWMPI 2013 in sunny Berkeley we are pleased to host the 4th International Workshop on Magnetic Particle Imaging in Berlin, Germany's innovative and vibrant capital. Demonstrating the growing interest in MPI, participants from 15 different countries will present more than 100 contributions (34 oral, 4 keynote speeches and 63 posters) spread across sessions for 'Magnetic Particle Imaging', 'Imaging Technology and Safety', 'Modelling, Simulation, Reconstruction and Sequences', 'MPI Theory, Relaxometry, Magnetometry', 'Magnetic Nanoparticles and Tracer Materials' and 'Medical Applications'.

As chairs of the workshop we would like to thank the members of the program committee:
G. Adam, UKE Hamburg; C. Alexiou, University of Erlangen; J. Barkhausen, UKSH Lübeck;
V. Behr, University of Würzburg; J. Bulte, John Hopkins University, Baltimore;
S. M. Conolly, University of California, Berkeley; O. Dössel, University of Karlsruhe;
S. Dutz, IPHT Jena; M. Ferguson, University of Washington; D. Finas, EVKB Bielefeld;
B. Gleich, Philips Technology GmbH, Hamburg; P. W. Goodwill, University of California, Berkeley;
M. Griswold, Case Western Reserve University, Cleveland; U. Häfeli, University of British Columbia, Vancouver; J. Haueisen, Ilmenau University of Technology; M. Heidenreich, Bruker BioSpin, Ettlingen;
U. Heinen, Bruker BioSpin, Ettlingen; Y. Ishihara, Meiji University; P. Jakob,University of Würzburg;
F. Kießling, University of Aachen; T. Knopp, Thorlabs, Lübeck; K. Krishnan, University of Washington;
F. Ludwig, TU Braunschweig; M. Magnani, University of Urbino; S. Odenbach, TU Dresden; Q. Pankhurst, Davy-Faraday Research Laboratory, London; U. Pison, Charité Berlin;
J. Rahmer, Philips Technology GmbH, Hamburg; A. Samia, Case Western Reserve University, Cleveland; E. U. Saritas, University of California, Berkeley; M. Schilling, Braunschweig University of Technology; I. Schmale, Philips Technology GmbH, Hamburg; J. Schnorr, Charité Berlin;
G. Schuetz, Bayer HealthCare, Berlin; M. Taupitz, Charité Berlin; B. ten Haken, University of Twente;
L. Trahms, PTB Berlin; J. Weaver, Dartmouth-Hitchcock Medical Center, Lebanon;
J. Weizenecker, Karlsruhe University of Applied Sciences; H. Weller, CAN Hamburg;
F. Wiekhorst, PTB Berlin

Most importantly, we would like to extend our gratitude to the members of the local organization teams for their tremendous efforts and work, and to Philips Healthcare, Bruker BioSpin, Bayer Healthcare Pharmaceuticals, MagQu Co. Ltd., be Berlin, GE Healthcare, Life Science Nord, Physikalisch-Technische Bundesanstalt (PTB), TSB Technologiestiftung Berlin, Imaging Netzwerk Berlin (INB), GruenderCUBE, Topass GmbH, Schuetz Brandcom, nanoPET Pharma GmbH, DGBMT, IEEE, EMB, Charité, and Hotel INDIGO for their support of the workshop.

We are already looking forward to next years' IWMPI that brings us to Istanbul.

Thorsten M. Buzug and Jörn Borgert

Lübeck and Hamburg, March 2014

Contents

TALKS

MAGNETIC PARTICLE IMAGING I

Challenges in the Application of Magnetic Particle Imaging
Dr. Bernhard Gleich 2

Integrated TWMPI-MRI Hybrid Scanner
Peter Klauer, *Patrick Vogel, Martin A. Rückert, Walter H. Kullmann, Peter M. Jakob, Volker C. Behr* 3

Spin Electronics Based Sensors for Low Frequency Magnetic Signal Detection
Fermon Claude, *Pannetier-Lecoeur Myriam, Lebras-Jasmin Guénaelle* 5

Drive-Field Decoupling and Control Network for Magnetic Particle Imaging
Jochen Franke, *Claas Bontus, Bernhard Gleich, Ulrich Heinen, Frederic Jaspard, Tobias Knopp, Wolfgang Ruhm, Michael Heidenreich, Thorsten M. Buzug* 6

X-space Image Reconstruction Algorithm with Optimized 2D/3D DC Recovery
Justin Konkle, *Patrick Goodwill, Michael Lustig, Kuan Lu, Steven Conolly* 7

IMAGING TECHNOLOGY AND SAFETY

Imaging of MNP using a Second Harmonic of Magnetization with DC Bias Field
Saburo Tanaka, *Hayaki Murata, Tomoya Ohishi, Yoshimi Hatsukade, Yi Zhang, Herng-Er Horng, Shu-Hsien Liao, Hong-Chang Yang* 10

Water-cooled Two-axis Rigid Excitation Coil Assembly
Patrick Goodwill, *Kuan Lu, Bo Zheng, Steven Conolly* 12

Considerations on Safety Limits for Magnetic Fields used in Magnetic Particle Imaging
Olaf Doessel, *Julia Bohnert* 14

MPI Safety in the View of MRI Safety Norms
Ingo Schmale, *Bernhard Gleich, Jürgen Rahmer, Claas Bontus, Joachim Schmidt, Jörn Borgert* 15

Strategies for Fast MPI within the Limits Determined by Nerve Stimulation
J. Rahmer, *J. Borgert, B. Gleich, I. Schmale, C. Bontus, J. Gressmann, C. Vollertsen* 16

MODELLING, SIMULATION, RECONSTRUCTION & SEQUENCES

UC Berkeley Innovations in MPI Hardware, Image Reconstruction, and Nanoparticles, with Application to Quantitative *In Vivo* Stem Cell Tracking
Prof. Steven Conolly 18

Compressed Sensing and Sparse Reconstruction in MPI
Anselm von Gladiß, *Mandy Ahlborg, Tobias Knopp, Thorsten M. Buzug* 19

Reconstruction Enhancement By Using Frequency Domain filters
Alexander Weber, *Jürgen Weizenecker, Jochen Franke, Ulrich Heinen, Michael Heidenreich, Wolfgang Ruhm, Thorsten Buzug* 21

A Phenomenological Description of the MPS-Signal Using a Model for the Field Dependence of the Effective Relaxation Time
Daniel Schmidt, *Florian Palmetshofer, David Heinke, Uwe Steinhoff, Frank Ludwig* 23

Debye-Based Frequency-Domain Magnetization Model for Magnetic Nanoparticles and its Application to Viscosity-Dependent MPS Measurements
Thilo Wawrzik, *Meinhard Schilling, Frank Ludwig* 25

MPI THEORY, RELAXOMETRY, MAGNETOMETRY

Simultaneous Reconstruction and Resolution Enhancement for Magnetic Particle Imaging
Osama A. Omer, *Hanne Wojtczyk, Thorsten M. Buzug* 28

Field Dependent Characteristic Timescales for Magnetic Nanoparticle Rotations
Daniel B. Reeves, *John B. Weaver* 30

Dependence of Brownian and Néel Relaxation Times on Magnetic Field Strength
Robert J. Deissler 31

Handheld Differential Magnetometry With a Split Coil Geometry
Sebastiaan Waanders, *Tasio Oderkerk, Martijn Visscher, Erik Krooshoop, Bennie ten Haken* 32

MAGNETIC NANOPARTICLES & TRACER MATERIALS

Optimized Tracers for MPI: Progress and Challenges
Prof. Kannan Krishnan 36

Dynamic Magnetic Behaviour of DDM128 in Agarose Gel, Gelatine and Sugar Matrix
Dietmar Eberbeck, *Lutz Trahms* 37

Dependence of Temperature Probing on Taylor's Expansion of Langevin Function Using Magnetic Nanoparticles in DC Field
Ling Jiang, *Wenzhong Liu, Jing Zhong, Pu Zhang* 38

Synthetic Approaches for Iron Oxide Nanoparticles Suitable as Tracer for Magnetic Particle Imaging
Andreas Ide, *Farnoosh Roohi, Hubertus Pietsch, Gunnar Schuetz* 40

Perpendicular Magnetic Particle Imaging, pMPI
John B. Weaver 41

MAGNETIC NANOPARTICLES & TRACER MATERIALS II

Optimized MPI Tracers Perform Well Over a Range of Excitation Field Conditions
R. Matthew Ferguson, *Scott J. Kemp, Amit P. Khandhar, Kannan M. Krishnan* 44

Hydrodynamic Fractionation to Enhance MPI Performance of Resovist®
Norbert Löwa, *Patrick Knappe, Dietmar Eberbeck, Andreas F. Thuenemann, Lutz Trahms* 46

Magnetic Characterisation of Clustered Core Magnetic Nanoparticles for MPI
Nicole Gehrke, *David Heinke, Dietmar Eberbeck, Frank Ludwig, Thilo Wawrzik, Christian Kuhlmann, Andreas Briel* 48

Tuning Magnetic Dipolar Interaction for Enhancing Magnetic Particle Imaging Performance
Subhasis Sarangi 50

Tuning Surface Coatings of Optimized Magnetite Nanoparticle Tracers for *In Vivo* MPI
Amit P. Khandhar, *R. Matthew Ferguson, Hamed Arami, Scott J. Kemp, Kannan M. Krishnan* 51

MEDICAL APPLICATIONS

Challenges for MPI: What are the Requirements a New Diagnostic Tool Must Meet?
Prof. Matthias Taupitz 54

Stem Cell Vitality Assessment Using Magnetic Particle Spectroscopy
Florian Fidler, *Maria Steinke, Alexander Kraupner, Cordula Gruettner, Karl-Heinz Hiller, Andreas Briel, Fritz Westphal, Heike Walles, Peter Michael Jakob* 55

Magnetic Particle Imaging (MPI): Visualization and Quantification of Vascular Stenosis Phantoms
Julian Haegele, *Jürgen Rahmer, Robert Duschka, Catharina Schaecke, Nicolaos Panagiotopoulos, Julia Tonak, Jörn Borgert, Joerg Barkhausen, Florian M. Vogt* 57

Time-Evolution Contrast of Target MRI Using Antibody Functionalized Magnetic Nanoparticles: An Animal Model
S.Y. Yang, *H.E. Horng, J.J. Chieh, C.C. Wu, K.W. Huang, H.C. Yang* 59

In Vivo MPI Neural Cell Monitoring in the Rat Brain
Bo Zheng, *Tandis Vazin, Patrick Goodwill, David Schaffer, Steven Conolly* 61

MAGNETIC PARTICLE IMAGING II

Flow Assessment from *In Vitro* and *In Silico* Dynamic MPI Data
Romain Lacroix, *Jürgen Rahmer, Oliver M. Weber, Hernan G. Morales, Sherif Makram-Ebeid* 64

Two Dimensional Magnetic Particle Imaging with a Dynamic Field Free Line Scanner
Klaas Bente, *Matthias Weber, Matthias Gräser, Mandy Ahlborg, Anselm v. Gladiss, Ksenija Gräfe, Gael Bringout, Marlitt Erbe, Timo F. Sattel, Thorsten M. Buzug* 66

Concept of a Generator for the Selection- and Focus Field of a Clinical MPI Scanner
Claas Bontus, *Bernhard Gleich, Bernd David, Oliver Mende, Jörn Borgert* 67

Ultra High Resolution MPI
Patrick Vogel, *Martin A. Rückert, Peter M. Jakob, Volker C. Behr* 68

LIST OF POSTERS

MAGNETIC PARTICLE IMAGING

P01 Efficient Gradient Fields in Magnetic Particle Imaging – From One Dimension to Multiple Dimensions
Christian Kaethner, Tobias Knopp, Mandy Ahlborg, Timo F. Sattel, Thorsten M. Buzug ... 72

P02 Measurement of System Functions with Extended Field-of-View
Nils Dennis Nothnagel, Javier Sanchez-Gonzalez, Aleksi Halkola, Jürgen Rahmer ... 74

P03 Projected Traveling Wave MPI
Patrick Vogel, Martin A. Rückert, Peter Klauer, Walter H. Kullmann, Peter M. Jakob, Volker C. Behr ... 75

P04 Superspeed Traveling Wave MPI
Patrick Vogel, Martin A. Rückert, Peter Klauer, Walter H. Kullmann, Peter M. Jakob, Volker C. Behr ... 77

P05 Setup and Validation of an MPI Signal Chain for a Drive Field Frequency of 150 kHz
T. F. Sattel, O. Woywode, J. Weizenecker, J. Rahmer, B. Gleich, J. Borgert ... 79

P06 Towards a Holistic MPI Signal Detection Using a Field Cancelation Local Receive Coil Topology
Volkmar Schulz, Max Mahlke, Simon Hubertus, Fabian Kiessling, Marcel Straub ... 80

P07 Experimental Demonstration of Multichannel Magnetic Particle Imaging for Improved Resolution
Kuan Lu, Patrick Goodwill, Steven Conolly ... 82

P08 Asymmetric Scanner Design for Unlimited Patient Access in Magnetic Particle Imaging
Christian Kaethner, Ksenija Gräfe, Mandy Ahlborg, Gael Bringout, Timo F. Sattel, Thorsten M. Buzug ... 84

P09 Initial Results of the First Commercial Preclinical MPI Scanner
Jochen Franke, Ulrich Heinen, Alexander Weber, Nicoleta Baxan, Ute Molkentin, Sarah Hermann, Wolfgang Ruhm, Michael Heidenreich ... 86

IMAGING TECHNOLOGY AND SAFETY

P10 Ultra-Low Field MRI Technology Using High-Temperature Superconductor SQUID
Junichi Hatta, Shingo Tsunaki, Masaaki Yamamoto, Yoshimi Hatsukade, Saburo Tanaka ... 88

P11 Experimental Evaluation of Iterative Reconstruction Method for Time-Correlation Magnetic Particle Imaging
Hiroki Tsuchiya, Takumi Homma, Syota Shimizu, Yasutoshi Ishihara ... 90

P12 System Matrix Recording and Phantom Measurements with a Single-Sided MPI Scanner
Ksenija Gräfe, Gael Bringout, Matthias Graeser, Timo Sattel, Thorsten M. Buzug ... 92

P13 Construction of a Multi-Dimensional Transmit Field Generator and Receive Coil Setup
Matthias Gräser, Timo Sattel, Thorsten M. Buzug ... 94

P14 Challenges of Stable MRI Data Acquisition Using the Preclinical MPI-MRI Hybrid System
Jochen Franke, Sascha Köhler, Franek Hennel, Alexander Weber, Ulrich Heinen, Wolfgang Ruhm, Michael Heidenreich, Thorsten M. Buzug ... 96

P15 Automated Derivation of Sub-Volume System Functions for 3D MPI with Fast Continuous Focus Field Variation
J. Rahmer, B. Gleich, C. Bontus, J. Schmidt, I. Schmale, J. Borgert, O. Woywode, A. Halkola, T. M. Buzug ... 97

P16 Shielded Drive Coils for a Rabbit Sized FFL Scanner
Gael Bringout, Mandy Ahlborg, Matthias Gräser, Christian Kaethner, Jan Stelzner, Wiebke Tenner, Hanne Wojtczyk, Thorsten M. Buzug ... 98

P17 Technical Aspects of a Two Dimensional Rotatable Field Free Line Imager for Magnetic Particle Imaging
Matthias Weber, Klaas Bente, Matthias Gräser, Mandy Ahlborg, Anselm v. Gladiss, Ksenija Gräfe, Gael Bringout, Marlitt Erbe, Timo F. Sattel, Thorsten M. Buzug ... 99

P18 Magnetic Particle Imaging with High-T_c Based SQUID Sensor
Hong-Chang Yang, Herng-Er Horng, Shu-Hsien Liao, Jen-Je Chieh ... 100

P19 MPI Based Hybrid Design for Actuation and Monitoring of Magnetic Nanoparticles for Targeted Drug Delivery
Ammar Mahmood, Mohammad Dadkhah, Jungwon Yoon ... 101

MODELLING, SIMULATION, RECONSTRUCTION & SEQUENCES

P20   Comparison of x-Space and Chebyshev Reconstruction in Magnetic Particle Imaging
Mandy Ahlborg, *Tobias Knopp, Thorsten M. Buzug* 104

P21   Simulation Study on Iterative Reconstruction Method for Time-Correlation Magnetic Particle Imaging with Continuous Trajectory Scan
Shota Shimizu, *Takumi Homma, Hiroki Tsuchiya, Yasutoshi Ishihara* 106

P22   Trajectory Analysis Using Patches for Magnetic Particle Imaging
Patryk Szwargulski, *Mandy Ahlborg, Christian Kaethner, Thorsten M. Buzug* 108

P23   Simulating and Modeling Relaxation Effects in Magnetic Particle Imaging
Martin A. Rückert, *Patrick Vogel, Peter M. Jakob, Volker C. Behr* 110

P24   Evaluation of Quantity and Linearity with regard to Tikhonov Regularization, Number of Iterations and Selection of Frequency Components in the MPI Reconstruction Process
Alexander Weber, *Jochen Franke, Jürgen Weizenecker, Ulrich Heinen, Michael Heidenreich, Wolfgang Ruhm, Thorsten M. Buzug* 112

P25   Magnetic Particles Image Reconstruct through Jacobi Singular Value Decomposition
Su Rijian, *Guo Gongbing, Zhang Qiuwen, Gan Yong, Huang Zhen, Zhong Jing, Du Zhongzhou* 113

P26   A Flexible and Modular MPI Simulation Framework and Its Use in Modelling a μMPI
Marcel Straub, *Fabian Kiessling, Volkmar Schulz* 114

P27   Magnetic Field Simulation Toolbox for MPI Modeling
Waldemar T. Smolik, *Przemysław R. Wróblewski, Jan Szyszko* 116

MPI THEORY, RELAXOMETRY, MAGNETOMETRY

P28   Rotational Drift Spectroscopy for Magnetic Particle Ensembles
Martin A. Rückert, *Patrick Vogel, Anna Vilter, Walter H. Kullmann, Peter M. Jakob, Volker C. Behr* 120

P29   Simulating the Signal Generation of Rotational Drift Spectroscopy
Martin A. Rückert, *Patrick Vogel, Thomas Kampf, Walter H. Kullmann, Peter M. Jakob, Volker C. Behr* ... 122

P30   Magnetic Particle Spectroscopy to Determine the Magnetic Drug Targeting Efficiency of Different Magnetic Nanoparticles in a Flow Phantom
Patricia Radon, *Maik Liebl, Nadine Pömpner, Marcus Stapf, Frank Wiekhorst, Kurt Gitter, Ingrid Hilger, Stefan Odenbach, Lutz Trahms* 124

P31   Framework to Characterize MPI Tracers in Terms of Achievable Resolution, FOV and Spectral Detection Limit
Florian Palmetshofer, *Daniel Schmidt, Uwe Steinhoff* 126

P32   Optimization of Inhomogeneous Excitation Fields in Magnetorelaxometry Imaging of Magnetic Nanoparticles
Daniel Baumgarten, *Friedemann Braune, Roland Eichardt, Jens Haueisen* 128

P33   Dual Models of Scanning SQUID Biosusceptometry for Simultaneous Functional Images of Magnetic- Nanoparticles Distribution and Structural Images of Animal Bodies
H.E. Horng, *J. J. Chieh, K. W. Huang, C. Y. Hong, H. C. Yang* 130

P34   Magnetic Particle Imaging Using Second and Third Harmonic of Magnetization Response
Hong-Chang Yang, *Herng-Er Horng, Shu-Hsien Liao, Jen-Je Chieh* 131

P35   DC and AC Magnetic Susceptometry of Superparamagnetic Fluids and Flims by Optical Polarimetry
Philipp Aebischer, *Victor Lebedev, Antoine Weis* 132

P36   Spatially Resolved *In Vitro* Spion Magnetorelaxometry Using Atomic Magnetometers
Victor Lebedev, *Simone Colombo, Vladimir Dolgovskiy, Antoine Weis* 134

MAGNETIC NANOPARTICLES & TRACER MATERIALS

P37 Tracers for Magnetic Particle Imaging Consisting of Agglomerated Single Cores
Silvio Dutz, Norbert Buske, Norbert Löwa, Dietmar Eberbeck, Lutz Trahms 138

P38 Ferrofluids of Modified Ultra Small Magnetic Particles for Application in Theranostics
Norbert Buske, Natascha Schelero, Lars Dähne, Ines Krumbein, Jürgen R. Reichenbach, Silvio Dutz 140

P39 Bacterial Magnetosomes as a New Type of Biogenic MPI Tracers
Alexander Kraupner, David Heinke, Rene Uebe, Dietmar Eberbeck, Nicole Gehrke, Dirk Schueler, Andreas Briel 141

P40 The Impact of the Size Distribution of Nanoparticles in Magnetic Nanothermometry
Zhongzhou Du, Wenzhong Liu, Jing Zhong, Paulo Cesar Morais 143

P41 AC Magnetization Spectrum for Magnetic Nanoparticle Temperature Estimation: An Investigation of AC Applied Magnetic Field
Zhongzhou Du, Wenzhong Liu, Jing Zhong, Ming Zhou 145

P42 Comparison of Temperature Estimation Employing Magnetization and Inverse Susceptibility of Magnetic Nanoparticles in DC Field
Ling Jiang, Wenzhong Liu, Jing Zhong 147

P43 Continuously Manufactured Magnetic Polymersomes as Potential Theranostic Tools in Nanomedicine
Regina Bleul, Norbert Löwa, Raphael Thiermann, Urs O. Häfeli, Gernot U. Marten, Michael J. House, Timothy G. St. Pierre, Lutz Trahms, Michael Maskos 149

P44 Evaluation of Hysteresis Loop and Magnetic Relaxation Time of Magnetic Nanoparticles Under Alternating Magnetic Field
Satoshi Ota, Kosuke Nakamura, Asahi Tomitaka, Tsutomu Yamada, Yasushi Takemura 151

P45 Drive Field Frequency Dependent MPI Performance of Single Core Magnetite Nanoparticles
Christian Kuhlmann, Amit P. Khandhar, R. Matthew Ferguson, Scott J. Kemp, Kannan M. Krishnan, Thilo Wawrzik, Meinhard Schilling, Frank Ludwig 152

P46 Structural Characterization of Clustered Core Iron Oxide Nanoparticles for MPI by Small Angle X-Ray Scattering
Nicole Gehrke, Stefan Wellert, David Heinke, Andreas Briel, Dietmar Eberbeck 154

P47 Production of Monosized Magnetic Microspheres by Microfluidic Flow Focusing
Mehrdad Bokharaei, Silvio Dutz, Urs O. Häfeli 156

P48 Viscosity Affected Determination of Iron Concentration of MPI Tracers Based on µCT
Christina Debbeler, Kerstin Lüdtke-Buzug 157

P49 Development of Superparamagnetic Surface Coatings
Kerstin Lüdtke-Buzug, Christina Debbeler 158

P50 Novel Developed Superparamagnetic Dextran Coated Iron Oxide Nanoparticles (SPION) as a Potential Tool for HNSCC Tumor Cell Detection and Its Influence on the Biological Properties
Ralph Pries, Antje Lindemann, Kerstin Lüdtke-Buzug, Barbara Wollenberg 159

P51 A Size-Resolved Analysis of Encapsulated Iron Oxide Nanoparticles and RESOVIST®
Jan Niehaus, Sören Becker, Christian Schmidtke, Arthur Feld, Horst Weller 160

P52 Influence on MPI Properties of Multilayer Iron Oxide Core
Hugo Groult, Nils Dennis Nothnagel, Jesus Ruiz-Cabello, Fernando Herranz 161

P53 Comparison of Some Magnetic Multicomponent Nanoparticles for Biomedical Applications
Nurcan Dogan, Ayhan Bingölbali, M. Asilturk, Z. Yeşil 162

P54 Measuring Dipolar Interactions and Magnetic Correlations in Self-Assembled Nanoparticle Superstructures with Electron Holography
Marco Beleggia, Miriam Varon, Tekeshi Kasama, Richard J Harrison, Rafal E Dunin-Borkowski, Victor F Puntes, Cathrine Frandsen 163

MEDICAL APPLICATIONS

P55 SPIO Detection and Distribution in Biological Tissue - a Murine MPI-SNLB Breast Cancer Model
Dominique Finas, Kristin Baumann, Lotta Sydow, Katja Heinrich, Achim Rody, Ksenija Gräfe, Kerstin Lüdtke-Buzug, Thorsten M. Buzug ... 166

P56 Magnetic Iron Nanoparticles as Useful Tool for Directing and Detecting Cells in Regenerative Medicine
Marc Schwarz, **Philipp Tripal**, Stefan Lyer, Frank Wiekhorst, Tobias Engelhorn, Tobias Struffert, Arnd Doerfler, Lutz Trahms, Christoph Alexiou ... 167

P57 Use of Red Blood Cells to Prolong the *In Vivo* Life Span of Iron-Based Contrast Agents for MRI and MPI
Mauro Magnani, Antonella Antonelli, Carla Sfara, Jürgen Rahmer, Bernhard Gleich, Jörn Borgert ... 168

P58 Time Behavior of Ferrofluids Under Liquid Stream Conditions in Magnetic Drug Targeting Applications: Simulation and Experimental Investigation
I. Slabu, A. Röth, G. Guentherodt, T. Schmitz-Rode, M. Baumann ... 170

P59 Toward Localized *In Vivo* Biomarker Concentration Measurements
John B. Weaver, Daniel Reeves, Yipeng Shi, Alexander Hartov, Barjor Gimi, Krishnamurthy V. Nemani ... 171

P60 FDTD Analysis of Electromagnetically Induced Heating and Bio-heat Transfer for Magnetic Fluid Hyperthermia
Wu Lei, Cheng Jingjing, Liu Wenzhong ... 173

P61 Visualization of Magnetic Nanoparticles in the Tumour Area after Intra-Arterial or Intra-Tumoural Application
Stefan Lyer, **Marc Schwarz**, Tobias Engelhorn, Tobias Struffert, Arnd Dörfler, Christoph Alexiou ... 174

P62 Optimization of Oncolytic Virus/Magnetic-Nanoparticle-Complexes for Tumor Therapy
Florian Wille, Olga Mykhaylyk, Jennifer Altomonte, Juliane Dworniczak, Isabella Almstätter, Ernst Rummeny, Oliver Ebert, Christian Plank, Rickmer Braren ... 175

P63 MR Imaging of a SPIO-Labeled Pathogen *In Vivo*: Distribution of Parasitic Protozoan Entamoeba Histolytica in the Liver of a Mouse Model at 7T
Harald Ittrich, Thomas Ernst, Hannah Bernin, Gerhard Adam, Hannelore Lotter ... 177

Session 1

Magnetic Particle Imaging I

Chairs: V. Behr, F. Ludwig

Keynote

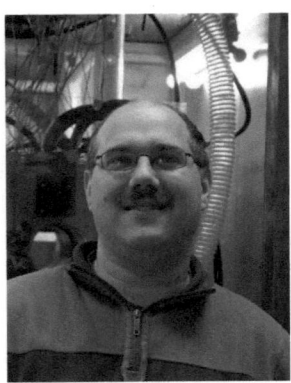

Dr. Bernhard Gleich

Philips Technologie GmbH, Innovative Technologies,
Research Laboratories, Hamburg, Germany

Challenges in the Application of Magnetic Particle Imaging

INTEGRATED TWMPI-MRI HYBRID SCANNER

Peter Klauer[1,3], Patrick Vogel[1,2,3], Martin A. Rückert[1,3], Walter H. Kullmann[3],
Peter M. Jakob[1,2], Volker C. Behr[1]

[1]Department of Experimental Physics 5 (Biophysics), University of Würzburg, Germany
[2]Research Center for Magnetic Resonance Bavaria e.V. (MRB), Würzburg, Germany
[3]Institute of Medical Engineering, University of Applied Sciences Würzburg-Schweinfurt, Germany

Magnetic Particle Imaging (MPI) was firstly presented in 2005 [1]. It is based on the nonlinear response of ferromagnetic material and the fact that the magnetization saturates at sufficiently high magnetic fields. In contrast to Magnetic Resonance Imaging (MRI), MPI directly detects the concentration and distribution of superparamagnetic iron-oxide nanoparticles (SPIOs) without any background of any tissue. To overcome this issue a Traveling Wave MPI (TWMPI) device [2] was combined with a low field MRI scanner [3] to show the possibility of a hybrid scanner, containing both imaging modalities in the same device [4]. The hardware of both separate approaches should be improved and optimized to reach higher fields and a higher resolution especially for the MRI measurement [5].

The TWMPI scanner works with a novel gradient design, the dynamic linear gradient array (dLGA), which can generate and move the required field free points (FFP) linearly along the symmetry axis. The dLGA contains 20 single copper coil elements, which can be driven individually (fig. 1 (a)). For the TWMPI measurement the traveling wave approach is used (fig 1 (b)). The dLGA can also be used for the generation of a homogeneous B_0 field required for the MRI. For that the controlling of the dLGA must be changed. For a desired B_0 field of about 235 mT (10 MHz ([^{1}H]) a current at the coil elements of about 135-200 A is required, which is provided by a customized amplifier (fig. 1 (c)). The simulation of the magnetic field (fig. 1 (d)) with the MRI current settings shows a homogeneous field (fig. 1 (e)) over the half of the scanner (about 60 mm). In a first test the stability of the current controller could be tested up to 135 A for the B_0 field generation with the dLGA

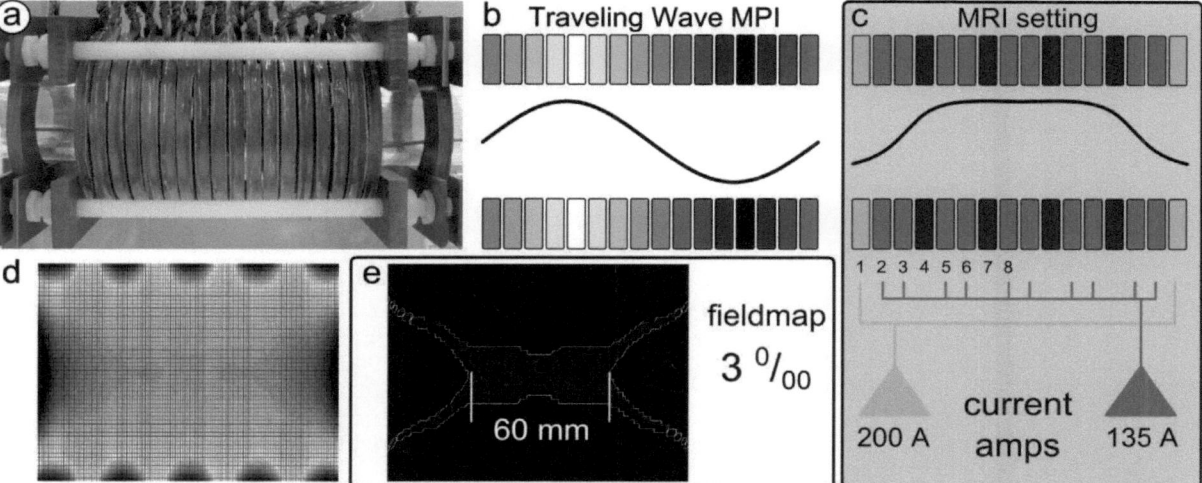

Fig. 1 (a) Dynamic linear gradient array (dLGA) contains several individually accessible coils. **(b)** Traveling wave mode for MPI measurement. **(c)** Current settings for the MRI measurement: the outer elements are driven with 200 A, the gray coils with 135 A and the black ones are not required in the MRI mode. **(d)** Magnetic field simulation with the MRI current settings. **(e)** Field homogeneity inside the scanner (inhomogeneity <0.3 %)).

Corresponding Author: P. Klauer, Peter.Klauer@physik.uni-Würzburg.de

[1] B. Gleich, and J. Weizenecker, "Tomographic imaging using the nonlinear response of magnetic particles", Nature 435, 1214-1217, Jun. 2005.

[2] P. Vogel et al. „Traveling Wave Magnetic Particle Imaging", IEEE TMI, 2013, Doi: 10.1109/TMI.2013.2285472.

[3] K.P. Pruessmann, "Less is more", Nature, 455, 43, 2008.

[4] P. Vogel and S. Lother, et al. "MPI meets MRI", Proc. DGMP 2013, p. 132f., Köln, 2013 (DGMP Abstractband, 2013).

[5] J. Franke et al. "First hybrid MPI-MRI imaging system as integrated design for mice and rats: descripton of the instrumentation setup", Proc. IWMPI, Berkeley, 2013 (IEEE – IWMPI 2013).

Corresponding Author: P. Klauer, Peter.Klauer@physik.uni-Würzburg.de

SPIN ELECTRONICS BASED SENSORS FOR LOW FREQUENCY MAGNETIC SIGNAL DETECTION

Fermon Claude, Pannetier-Lecoeur Myriam, Lebras-Jasmin Guénaelle

Nanomagnetism and oxide laboratory CEA Saclay, Gif Sur Yvette, France

Tuned or untuned coils are currently used for the detection of MRI signals or MPI detection. They are very sensitive at high frequencies but suffer at low frequencies of a reduced performance due to the fact that they detect the derivative over time of the flux. Alternative detection schemes with magnetic sensors able to detect directly the flux are hence competitive for frequencies below 1MHz. In the last years, we have developed spin electronics based sensors either cooled at low temperature, either working at room temperature which present better detectivities than tuned coils for frequencies below 300kHz. Low temperature sensors are using a superconducting loop acting as a flux to field transformer [1] which can be coupled to a cooled or room temperature pick-up loop. The detectivity is hence of about 10fT/sqrt(Hz) for frequencies down to 1kHz. Below 1kHz, the 1/f noise of spin electronics sensors decreases slightly the performances. At room temperature, the use of high performance ferrites as flux concentrators gives also detectivities in the same range above 10kHz. We will present device performances and some results applied to the case of on very low field (1-10mT/42-420kHz)) MRI. In particular we will show the first images obtained on in vivo tissues and the T1 and T2 values evaluated in the millitesla range [2].
This type of sensor could be also good candidates for Magnetic Particle Imaging [3], because they still exhibit very good sensitivity in the frequency range of few tens of kHz with a flat frequency response. We will evaluate the possible performances of such a detection scheme for Magnetic Particle Imaging experiment and discuss the advantages and drawbacks versus the tuned coil detection setups.

[1] Pannetier M, Fermon C, Le Goff G, Simola J and Kerr E(2004) Femtotesla magnetic field measurement with magnetoresistive sensors, Science, 304, 1648–50.

[2] Herreros, Q, Dyvorne, H, Campiglio P, Jasmin-Lebras G, Demonti A, Pannetier-Lecoeur M and Fermon C, Very low field magnetic resonance imaging with spintronics sensors, Rev. Sci. Instr. 84 (2013)

[3] Gleich B and Weizenecker J, Tomographic imaging using the nonlinear response of magnetic particles, Nature 435, 1214–1217 (2005).

Corresponding Author: F. Claude, claude.fermon@cea.fr

DRIVE-FIELD DECOUPLING AND CONTROL NETWORK FOR MAGNETIC PARTICLE IMAGING

Jochen Franke[1,5], Claas Bontus[2], Bernhard Gleich[2], Ulrich Heinen[1], Frederic Jaspard[3], Tobias Knopp[4], Wolfgang Ruhm[1], Michael Heidenreich[1], Thorsten M. Buzug[5]

[1]*Bruker BioSpin MRI GmbH, Ettlingen, Germany*
[2]*Philips Technologie GmbH, Hamburg, Germany*
[3]*Bruker BioSpin SAS, Wissembourg, France*
[4]*Thorlabs GmbH, Lübeck, Germany*
[5]*Institute of Medical Engineering, University of Lübeck, Germany*

Magnetic particle imaging (MPI) is a novel tracer-based imaging method allowing detection of the distribution of superparamagnetic iron oxide nanoparticles in vivo in three dimensions and in real time. For spatial encoding, MPI applies a static gradient field featuring a field-free point (FFP) at a unique position in space which is steered through the field-of-view (FoV) by means of three orthogonal homogenous AC drive-fields (DF), each with a dedicated frequency of around 25 kHz. The signal chain for each DF channel consists of a power amplifier, an analog band-pass filter, a matching network and a transmit coil. Each power amplifier A_i, i = x, y, z is fed with a sinusoidal three tone input signal at the three DF frequencies f_j, j = x, y, z represented by the Fourier coefficients $â_{i,j}$. The frequency components of the resulting currents in the DF coils, which can be measured inductively, are denoted as $ĉ_{i,j}$. A diagonal input matrix $â_{i,j}$, i.e. feeding only the main frequency f_i to the DF channel i, will in general not correspond to a diagonal output matrix $ĉ_{i,j}$ caused by inherent coil coupling in the DF system. To allow for stable excitation even for long calibrations scans as well as to ensure a rectangular FoV, two conditions of the resulting DF currents $ĉ_{i,j}$ have to be met:

- thermal drifts in the signal chain have to be actively compensated by controlling $ĉ_{i,j}$ (for i=j) in terms of stable amplitude and phase.
- all DF channels have to be decoupled, i.e. $ĉ_{i,j}$ should be zero for i≠j, as coupling leads directly to a sheared FoV.

Hence one has to exploit different approaches minimizing the DF coil current on the side frequencies in order to obtain a pure sinusoidal current in the DF coils: 1) optimized DF coil production that minimizes channel cross talk, 2) passive DF channel decoupling by means of a decoupling network, and 3) active cross talk compensation by means of DF current monitor and actively controlling of the input matrix $â_{i,j}$ to compensate for temporal changing residual couplings, i.e. for the side frequencies $ĉ_{i,j}$ with i≠j. To minimize the power requirements for A_i, all three approaches have to be combined, as active cross talk compensation alone would lead to enormous reactive power requirements mostly due to impedance mismatch of the signal chain at the side frequencies. In this work, an active control algorithm method for a 3D MPI scanner is presented to allow for drift compensation as well as active DF cross talk compensation using a numerical real-time PID controller. This method includes a three step measurement based determination of the band-structured 9x9 transfer matrix which maps $â_{i,j}$ to $ĉ_{i,j}$, while adequate PID control initialization minimizes the integral windup during the transient phase of the controller. The DF control algorithm has been evaluated experimentally on a 3D MPI scanner (BRUKER MPI 25/20F), where $ĉ_{i,j}$ were assessed for the raw DF system and the passively decoupled DF system both with and w/o the active DF cross talk compensation, where the amplitude control for $ĉ_{i,j}$ (for i=j) has been used in each case.

Acknowledgements: The authors thankfully acknowledge the financial support by the German Federal Ministry of Education and Research, FKZ 13N11088.

Corresponding Author: J. Franke, Jochen.Franke@bruker-BioSpin.de

X-SPACE IMAGE RECONSTRUCTION ALGORITHM WITH OPTIMIZED 2D/3D DC RECOVERY

Justin Konkle[1], Patrick Goodwill[1], Michael Lustig[1,2], Kuan Lu[1], Steven Conolly[1,2]

[1]Department of Bioengineering, University of California, Berkeley, USA
[2]Department of Electrical Engineering and Computer Science, Berkeley, USA

INTRODUCTION: Two reconstruction formulations have been demonstrated in Magnetic Particle Imaging: 'system function' reconstruction [1-3] and x-space reconstruction [3-5]. With the x-space image reconstruction method, we grid our received signal to the instantaneous position of the field free line or field free point [4-5]. However, any MPI reconstruction algorithm must estimate the fundamental signal, which is lost during direct-feedthrough filtering[4-5]. In a prior x-space approach, the DC component of the image was recovered by enforcing 1D image continuity between image stations (or partial FOVs) [5].
METHODS: Here, we propose a full 2D or 3D continuity algorithm to be used in conjunction with the x-space reconstruction method. The reconstruction optimization problem is then solved via regularized least squares. Prior to optimization, we grid partial field of view images, which become the input to our reconstruction problem.
RESULTS: In Figure 1, we showed the result of our reconstruction algorithm on simulated data. We created partial field of view images from the input image. We then removed the DC value along the x-axis and added noise. As noted in the error image, the algorithm was quite robust to noise and accurately recovered the image.
CONCLUSION: The x-space DC recovery algorithm allows 2D or 3D image reconstruction, with full DC recovery. 2D or 3D continuity is a tighter constraint and should offer physically robust a *priori* information.

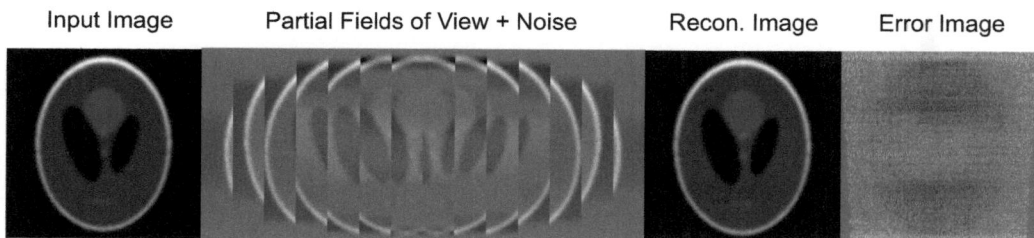

[1] B. Gleich and J. Weizenecker, "Tomographic imaging using the nonlinear response of magnetic particles.," Nature, vol. 435, no. 7046, pp. 1214-7, Jun. 2005.

[2] J. Rahmer, J. Weizenecker, B. Gleich, and J. Borgert, "Analysis of a 3-D system function measured for magnetic particle imaging.," IEEE Trans. Med. Imaging, vol. 31, no. 6, pp. 1289-99, Jun. 2012.

[3] J. Rahmer, J. Weizenecker, B. Gleich, and J. Borgert, "Signal encoding in magnetic particle imaging: properties of the system function.," BMC Med. Imaging, vol. 9, no. 1, p. 4, Jan. 2009.

[4] P. W. Goodwill and S. M. Conolly, "The X-space formulation of the magnetic particle imaging process: 1-D signal, resolution, bandwidth, SNR, SAR, and magnetostimulation.," IEEE Trans. Med. Imaging, vol. 29, no. 11, pp. 1851-9, Nov. 2010.

[5] K. Lu, P. W. Goodwill, E. U. Saritas, B. Zheng, and S. M. Conolly, "Linearity and shift invariance for quantitative magnetic particle imaging.," IEEE Trans. Med. Imaging, vol. 32, no. 9, pp. 1565-75, Sep. 2013.

Corresponding Author: J. Konkle, jkonkle@berkeley.edu

Session 2

Imaging Technology and Safety

Chairs: O. Dössel, S. Conolly

IMAGING OF MNP USING A SECOND HARMONIC OF MAGNETIZATION WITH DC BIAS FIELD

Saburo Tanaka[1], Hayaki Murata[1], Tomoya Ohishi[1], Yoshimi Hatsukade[1], Yi Zhang[2], Herng-Er Horng[3], Shu-Hsien Liao[3], Hong-Chang Yang[4]

[1]*Department of Environmental and Life Sciences, Toyohashi University of Technology, Japan*
[2]*Peter Gruenberg Institute, Forschungszentrum Juelich, Germany*
[3]*National Taiwan Normal University, Taipei, Taiwan*
[4]*Kun Shan University, Tainan, Taiwan*

Magnetic particle imaging (MPI) introduced by Gleich and Weizenecker is based on utilizing the non-linear magnetic response M for detection of super-paramagnetic iron oxide nanoparticles (MNP) [1]. The excited M contains not only the fundamental excitation frequency ω_0 but also its harmonics when applying an ac excitation magnetic field $H_{ac} = H_0\sin(\omega_0 t)$. A number of magnetic readout methods have been developed to determine the MNP volume (or mass) for different application purposes, for example, immunoassay [2-4]. In the MNP detection and the MPI technique, the most commonly employed method is the detection of the odd harmonics of the M response. We invented a method to improve the detection sensitivity for the magnetization M of MNP. The M response of MNP to an applied magnetic field H (M–H characteristics) could be divided into a linear region and a saturation region, which are separated at a transition (or saturation) point H_k. The M value shows the saturation trend at the field larger than H_k. We define this point on M–H characteristics as FKP (Field Knee Point) as shown in Fig. 1(a). When applying an excitation AC magnetic field (H_{ac}) and an additional DC bias field $H_{dc} = H_k$, the second harmonic of M reaches the maximum due to the nonlinearity of the M–H characteristics. It is stronger than any other harmonics including a third harmonic [5]. The advantage of the use of the second harmonic response is that the response can be taken for even in small amplitude of H_{ac}. In the case of the conventional detection using a third harmonic, the amplitude of the H_{ac} must be larger than the threshold level, which is almost the same as H_k. The M response of MNP was systematically analyzed and experimentally proven. In order to prove our assumption above, we performed experiments using a high-concentration MNP sample (Resovist®, 27.8 mg/ml, 60 nm in dia., 70㎖) under different H_{ac} and H_{dc}. For the detection of the sample M responses, three solenoid coils were employed: coil L_{dc} was used to generate the DC static field H_{dc}, L_{ac} to generate the AC excitation field H_{ac} and L_d to detect the M responses of MNP sample. L_d consisted of two coils arranged differentially as a gradient pickup coil which reduced the influence of fundamental frequency ω_0 (5kHz x 2π), thus increasing the amplifier dynamic range. One of the two coils surrounded the sample to detect its M response. The three coils, L_{dc}, L_{ac} and L_d, were arranged coaxially. A high sensitive magnetic sensor device, High-Tc SQUID magnetometer was magnetically connected to the pickup coil to amplify the signal at low noise. Keeping the ac excitation field constant at $H_{ac} = 0.57$ mT$_{pp}/\mu_0$, the M response harmonics of sample vs. the H_{dc} variation between ± 30 mT/μ_0 were recorded in Fig. 1(b). In other words, the bias point was scanned in the range of $H_{dc} \approx \pm 30$mT/μ_0. As expected, the M maxima of second harmonic appeared at $H_{dc} = \pm H_k = \pm 2.5$ mT/μ_0, while the third harmonic reached a maximum at $H_{dc} = 0$. The half-widths of the maximums were estimated to be about 3.1 mT/μ_0. No significant difference of the half-widths between the second harmonic and the third harmonic was observed. The half-width with a gradient field decides the imaging resolution of x-space in MPI technique [1]. For 1-D imaging, two identical ring-shaped permanent magnets (f120 x f100 x 20t, Surface magnetic density: 0.4T) were prepared and set with a space of 80 mm so that it gives linear magnetic gradient field of 2.63 mT/mm in the rage of ±15 mm. All the coils of L_{dc}, L_{ac} and L_d were coaxially placed in the space of the ring magnets. As a phantom, a small plastic-made container of f ϕ2

Corresponding Author: S. Tanaka, tanakas@ens.tut.ac.jp

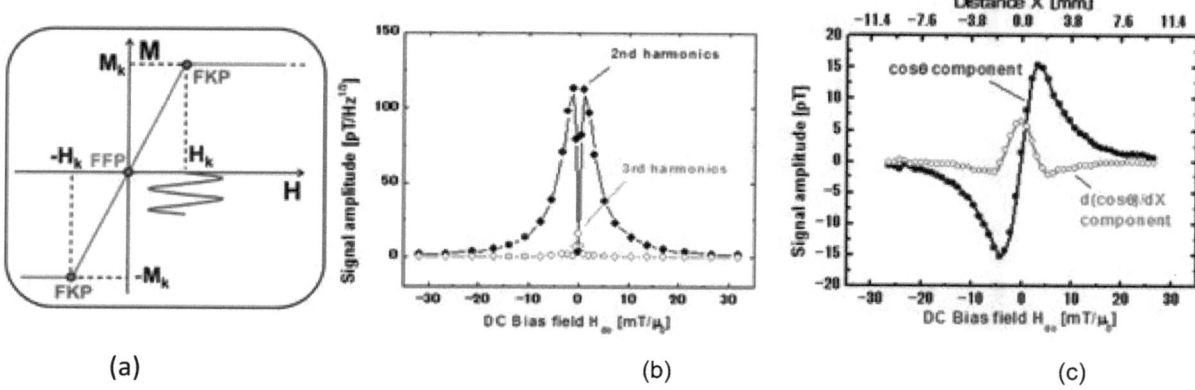

Fig.1. (a) Principle of the detection using a 2nd harmonic with dc bias field of H_k. (b) Dependence of M harmonics of sample on varying H_{dc}. (c) 1-D MPI image of MNP phantom.

x 3 mm filled with MNP solution (Resovist®) of 10ml was prepared and set in one of the two detection coils. The electronics for the imaging was the same as previous experiment, but the output of the SQUID amplifier was connected to a lock-in-amplifier to perform a phase sensitive detection. By changing the DC bias field H_{dc}, the bias point was scanned in the range of $H_{dc} \approx \pm 30\text{mT}/\mu_0$. The signal of $\cos\theta$ component from lock-in-amplifier was recorded; the recorded data was differentiated. Figure 1(c) shows the $\cos\theta$ component and its differentiated values as a function of the DC bias field. The DC bias field can be converted into the distance X, which is shown at the upper axis in the figure. The $\cos\theta$ component (solid circle) shows two peaks at FKP. The position of the MNP phantom must be located at the FFP, where the slope shows the maximum. However, since the position is not clear by this component, the differential component, $d(\cos\theta)/dX$ (open circle) was used to obtain the 1-D imaging. In the case it was easy to define the position of the MNP phantom by finding the peak of the component.

It was demonstrated that the second harmonic of M is stronger than any other harmonics. A high sensitive magnetic sensor device, SQUID magnetometer was used as a low noise amplifier. The detection method using a second harmonic was applied to MPI (Magnetic Particle Imaging). We could successfully demonstrate the 1D image of a column-shaped phantom filled with MNP.

This work was supported in part by Japanese-Taiwanese Cooperative Program on Bioelectronics.

[1] B. Gleich and J. Weizenecker, "Tomographic imaging using the nonlinear response of magnetic particles", Nature **435**, 1214 (2005).

[2] P. W. Goodwill, K. Lu, B. Zheng, and S. M. Conolly, "Optimizing magnetite nanoparticles for mass sensitivity in magnetic particle imaging", Rev. Sci. Instrum. **83**, 033708 (2012).

[3] K. Kriz, J. Gehrke, and D. Kriz, "Advancements toward magneto immunoassays", Biosensors Bioelectron. **13**, 817 (1998).

[4] H.-J. Krause, N. Wolters, Y. Zhang, A. Offenhaeussera, P. Miethe, M. H. F. Meyer, M. Hartmann, and M. Keusgen, "Magnetic particle detection by frequency mixing for immunoassay applications", J. Magn. Magn. Mater. **311**, 436 (2007).

[5] Yi Zhang, Hayaki Murata, Yoshimi Hatsukade and Saburo Tanaka, "Superparamagnetic nanoparticle detection using second harmonic of magnetization response", Rev. Sci. Instrum. **84**, 094702 (2013).

Corresponding Author: S. Tanaka, tanakas@ens.tut.ac.jp

WATER-COOLED TWO-AXIS RIGID EXCITATION COIL ASSEMBLY

Patrick Goodwill[1], Kuan Lu[1], Bo Zheng[1], Steven Conolly[1,2]

[1]Department of Bioengineering, University of California, Berkeley, USA
[2]Department of Electrical Engineering and Computer Science, Berkeley, USA

Introduction: The detection limit for MPI cell tracking is proportional to the velocity of scanning, which can be maximized for a particular excitation frequency by exciting at the magnetostimulation limit [1]. The magneto-stimulation limit for small animals is approximately 40 mT at 50 kHz in mice/rats [2], which can be challenging to achieve in imaging systems because of electrical power requirements [3]. Further, in a multi-axis transmit coil assembly, the power dissipation requirements can be demanding in the transverse axes since saddle and Helmholtz coils are less efficient than the solenoid coils used to produce axial fields.

Here we describe the construction of a rigid two-axis excitation coil assembly constructed for use in high-speed projection MPI imaging. We desired a rigid electromagnet to minimize any electromechanical distortion, which prevents us from using magnet wire in a liquid cooling bath. We constructed a prototype water-cooled two-axis transmit coil assembly capable of continuous excitation at kilowatt power levels with a 6.3 cm inner diameter using rigid copper tube. This coil assembly serves as a prototype for future coil sets that we aim to operate at the murine magneto-stimulation limits at over 5 kW power levels.

Methods: We constructed a medium-power transmit coil assembly for the Berkeley 7 T/m 3D MPI imager. The transmit coil set is capable of transmitting both transverse and axial to the imaging bore. The transverse excitation coil is a two-layer saddle coil CNC machined from plates of 1.6 mm copper plate using a home-built CNC router. After annealing and hammering into a saddle configuration, each of the four plates was insulated with Kapton insulation and soldered into a continuous circuit. The axial transmit coil is a water-cooled, hollow-core solenoid wound outer to the transverse coil. The entire assembly was then potted in heat conductive epoxy under vacuum.

Results: The coil is shown in Fig 1A. The transmit system achieved the design parameters of over 15 mT in both axes at 1.2 kW power levels (see Table 1). The electro-mechanical distortion of the coils during signal reception is also minimal (Fig. 1B). We also constructed transverse and axial receive coils in order to test the imaging functionality of the system. Images of a point source are shown in Fig. 1(C,D).

Coil orientation	Transmit Free Bore	Field Produced (peak-to-peak)	Receive Coil Sensitivity	Imaging Free Bore
Transverse (X axis)	6.3 cm	15 mT @ 1.2 kW	430 µT/A	5 cm
Axial (Z axis)	6.3 cm	17 mT @ 1.2 kW	800 µT/A	5 cm

Table 1: Two-channel transmit coil key parameters

Discussion: Here we demonstrated the construction and testing of a two-axis transmit coil assembly. The coil achieves the design goals of kilowatt power dissipation at 15 mT excitation strength across an imaging free bore of 5 cm (with receive coils), with both low noise and electromechanical distortion. This is the first demonstration of a rigid, water-cooled, two-axis transmit coil tailored for high-speed projection murine imaging.

Corresponding Author: P. Goodwill, goodwill@berkeley.edu

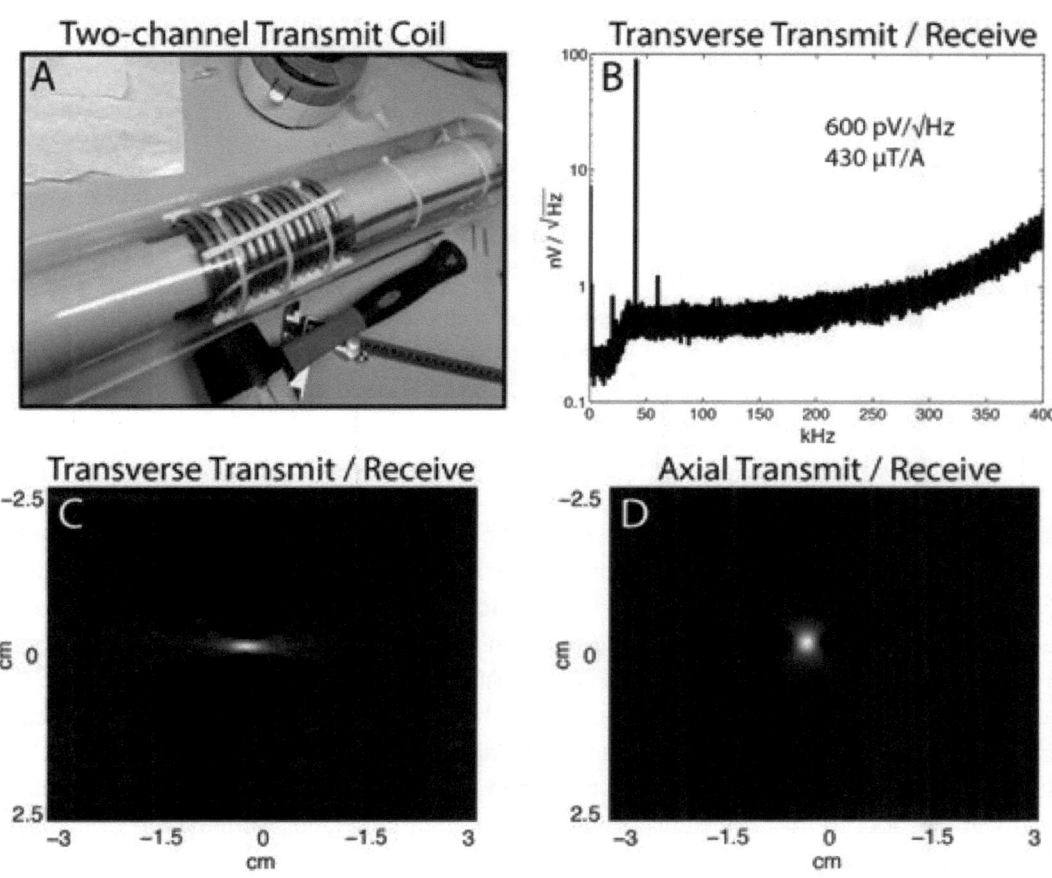

Fig 1: (A) Two-axis transmit coil before potting in heat conductive epoxy. (B) The noise and distortion spectrum of the transverse receive coil during signal reception. (C,D) Undeconvolved native image of a point source showing the expected "dog-bone" point spread function seen in x-space reconstruction. 1 μL Micromod-MIP tracer. 5 minute acquisition time, 5 cm x 4 cm x 6 cm FOV.

[1] J. Weizenecker, B. Gleich, J. Rahmer, H. Dahnke, and J. Borgert, "Three-dimensional real-time in vivo magnetic particle imaging.," Phys. Med. Biol., vol. 54, no. 5, pp. L1–L10, Mar. 2009.

[2] P. W. Goodwill and S. M. Conolly, "The X-space formulation of the magnetic particle imaging process: 1-D signal, resolution, bandwidth, SNR, SAR, and magnetostimulation.," IEEE Trans. Med. Imaging, vol. 29, no. 11, pp. 1851–9, Nov. 2010.

[3] J. Rahmer, B. Gleich, J. Schmidt, C. Bontus, I. Schmale, J. Kanzenbach, J. Borgert, O. Woywode, A. Halkola, J. Weizenecke, "Continuous Focus Field Variation for Extending the Imaging Range in 3D MPI" in S. Proceedings, Magnetic Particle Imaging, vol. 140. Berlin, Heidelberg: Springer Berlin Heidelberg, 2012.

Corresponding Author: P. Goodwill, goodwill@berkeley.edu

CONSIDERATIONS ON SAFETY LIMITS FOR MAGNETIC FIELDS USED IN MAGNETIC PARTICLE IMAGING

Olaf Doessel[1], Julia Bohnert[2]

[1]Institute of Biomedical Engineering, Karlsruhe Institute of Technology KIT, Karlsruhe, Germany
[2]now at ITK Engineering AG, Ruelzheim, Germany

For Magnetic Particle Imaging (MPI) magnetic fields in the frequency range of 10kHz to 100kHz are applied with amplitudes of 10mT to 100mT. Using larger fields will lead to a better signal to noise ratio and/or to a shorter acquisition time. Since the human body is conducting, these time varying magnetic fields will induce eddy currents that may lead to stimulation of muscle and heating of tissue. Annoying, painful or even dangerous effects may arise. Safety limits for the exposure of patients to magnetic fields in this frequency range have to be defined [1].

The frequency rage of 10kHz to 100kHz is not comprehensively explored yet in this respect. Below 10kHz the stimulation of nerves and muscle is dominating for the definition of thresholds. Various measurements of stimulation thresholds can be found in the literature. Often the current densities or the electric fields inside the muscle, that lead to the stimulation in these experiments, are not precisely known or not reported. Several articles propose simplified formulas that help to estimate the frequency dependency. Generally the threshold current density that is able to stimulate nerves or muscle is rising while increasing the frequency, but at the same time also the current density induced in the body goes up with frequency (keeping the amplitude of the magnetic field constant). This leads to a plateau of the threshold with respect to the amplitude of the applied magnetic field. Somewhere above 50kHz the beta-dispersion becomes important: the capacitance of the cell membrane leads to a short-cut for the currents and thus there is no "kick" to the transmembrane voltage any more.

Above the frequency range of about 25kHz the heating of the tissue through the eddy currents becomes very important. The important property in this respect is the Specific Absorption Rate SAR. SAR increases quadratically with frequency (keeping the amplitude of the magnetic field constant). Using Pennes bioheat equation the local rise of temperature can be calculated. Above 50kHz only a reduced duty cycle can prevent the tissue from being heated to temperatures that lead to damage.

This contribution cannot give a comprehensive answer to the question of adequate thresholds, but it will summarize (a) the application of basics of electromagnetic field theory to this problem, it will present (b) the most important published regulations in this field, it will (c) review the most important measurement results and formulas on stimulation thresholds for magnetic fields and it will (d) visualize current densities, SAR and temperature rise in a model of the human body using numerical field calculation.

[1] Olaf Doessel and Julia Bohnert, "Safety considerations for magnetic fields of 10 mT to 100 mT amplitude in the frequency range of 10 kHz to 100 kHz for magnetic particle imaging", Biomed Tech 2013; 58(6): 611-621

Corresponding Author: O. Doessel, olaf.doessel@kit.edu

MPI SAFETY IN THE VIEW OF MRI SAFETY NORMS

Ingo Schmale, Bernhard Gleich, Jürgen Rahmer, Claas Bontus, Joachim Schmidt, Jörn Borgert

Philips Technologie GmbH Innovative Technologies, Hamburg, Germany

Like in MRI, two physiological mechanisms limit the application of MPI to humans: PNS and SAR. For both, ample experience has been gained over years during the development of MRI. Human MPI is only at its beginning, with only limited dedicated experiments carried out so far, but can take advantage of the wealth of safety knowledge and norms from MRI.

The contribution will start by outlining the similarities and differences from MRI and MPI: RF, gradient, and B0 field versus Drive Field, Selection Field, and slow and fast Focus Fields. Then it will be shown how each of these terms influences PNS and SAR.

For PNS, the dependency of threshold as a function of frequency shall be discussed. It can be shown that early experimental results by Saritas et al. and our group are largely in line with MRI norms (e.g. IEC 60601-2-33). The relevance of differences shall be investigated: frequency, pulsed vs. continuous operation, trapezoidal vs. sinusoidal waveform, single vs. multi-frequency operation, the influence of spatially orthogonal simultaneous excitations, the influence of simultaneous application of fast-focus field and of drive field etc...

For SAR, the challenges of deriving a precise measure of dissipated power shall be discussed. Our experiments on Q-loading of the drive-field coils are presented and will be compared to numeric and analytic calculation for the used field generators. Both approaches include the effect of inhomogeneities of the magnetic field, with field increases near the field generator, but also with strongly decaying fields far off. As SAR is the ratio of power to weight, the question of what weight needs to be taken into account shall be discussed in light of the norm definitions of whole-body, partial-body, and local-tissue SAR.

Acknowledgement
This work was supported by the German Federal Ministry of Education and Research (BMBF grants FKZ 13N11086).

References

[1] Schmale et al., Human PNS and SAR Study in the Frequency Range from 24 to 162 kHz, 3rd IWM-PI, Berkeley, March 2013

[2] Saritas et al, Magnetostimulation Limits in Magnetic Particle Imaging, IEEE T on Medical Imaging, vol. 32, no. 9, Sept. 2013

Corresponding Author: I. Schmale, ingo.schmale@philips.com

STRATEGIES FOR FAST MPI WITHIN THE LIMITS DETERMINED BY NERVE STIMULATION

J. Rahmer[1], J. Borgert[1], B. Gleich[1], I. Schmale[1], C. Bontus[1], J. Gressmann[2], C. Vollertsen[2]

[1]*Philips Technologie GmbH Innovative Technologies, Research Laboratories, Hamburg, Germany*
[2]*Philips Medical Systems DMC GmbH, Hamburg, Germany*

Recent volunteer studies on nerve stimulation caused by the application of oscillating magnetic fields in the range between 0.5 and 160 kHz indicate that for clinical applications, MPI drive field amplitudes will be limited to values clearly below 10 mT [1, 2]. Compared to pre-clinical small-bore systems that apply field amplitudes up to 20 mT [3, 4], the reduced amplitudes result in a substantial reduction of the imaging volume encoded by the drive fields. For compensation, focus fields, which have been introduced to generate additional spatial shifts that extend the imaging volume [3], need to operate faster, while also respecting nerve stimulation thresholds.

In this contribution, strategies for fast spatial coverage are presented, which are based on a system design with three orthogonal drive fields, three orthogonal focus fields, and additional fast focus fields. To enable faster imaging and reduce nerve stimulation, the drive frequencies have been shifted from the range around 25 kHz to 150 kHz. Within the parameter space determined by applied selection field gradient strength, applicable field amplitudes and slew rates, trajectory density, and desired geometry of the imaging volume, different scenarios are evaluated with the aim to enable fast volumetric MPI in clinical applications.

The results indicate that within the limits imposed by nerve stimulation thresholds, hardware limitations, and rather low MPI-performance of currently available approved tracer materials, true real-time imaging at high resolution will not be feasible over large volumes (e.g. the whole heart), but will be restricted to sub-volumes, whose shape can be quite freely adapted to the anatomy of interest. Alternatively, real-time MPI of large volumes can be performed at reduced spatial resolution by scaling down the selection field gradient applied for spatial encoding. From the complementary information acquired at different spatial and temporal resolutions, synthetic real-time representations of larger volumes can be generated with high spatial resolution.

ACKNOWLEDGMENT

This work was supported by the German Federal Ministry of Education and Research (BMBF grant FKZ 13N11086).

[1] EU Saritas et al., "Magnetostimulation Limits in Magnetic Particle Imaging.", IEEE Transactions on Medical Imaging 32, no. 9 (September 2013): 1600–1610.

[2] I Schmale et al., "Human PNS and SAR Study in the Frequency Range from 24 to 162 kHz.", IEEE Proc. IWMPI 2013.

[3] B Gleich et al., "Fast MPI Demonstrator with Enlarged Field of View.", Proc. ISMRM, 18:218, 2010.

[4] J Franke et al., "First Hybrid MPI-MRI Imaging System as Integrated Design for Mice and Rats: Description of the Instrumentation Setup.", IEEE Proc. IWMPI 2013.

Corresponding Author: J. Rahmer, Jürgen.rahmer@philips.com

Session 3

Modelling, Simulation, Reconstruction & Sequenzes

Chairs: J. Weizenecker, B. Gleich

Keynote

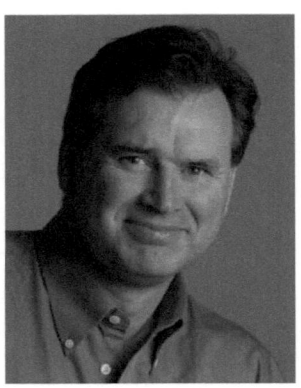

Prof. Steven Conolly

Bioengineering, and Electrical Engineering & Computer Sciences
University of California, Berkeley, USA

UC Berkeley innovations in MPI hardware, image reconstruction, and nanoparticles, with application to quantitative *in vivo* stem cell tracking

COMPRESSED SENSING AND SPARSE RECONSTRUCTION IN MPI

Anselm von Gladiß[1], Mandy Ahlborg[1], Tobias Knopp[2], Thorsten M. Buzug[1]

[1]Institute of Medical Engineering, Universität zu Lübeck, Germany
[2]THORLABS GmbH, Lübeck, Germany

The reconstruction of a particle concentration in Magnetic Particle Imaging (MPI) usually involves the solution of a linear system of equations [1]. The acquisition and storage of the system matrix is challenging in practice: The acquisition time is proportional to the discretisation of the field of view (FOV). Assuming optimistic conditions, the system matrix acquisition lasts about two days for a spatial grid containing 64x64x64 voxels. Such a system matrix has a memory size of about 300 GB and therefore, it cannot be stored in the main memory of the computer, which is necessary for the application of fast reconstruction algorithms. As it has been recently shown, the acquisition time of a system matrix can be reduced significantly using compressed sensing methods [2]. It suffices to undersample the system matrix by acquiring only 20 % of the voxels in the FOV [3]. These points are randomly selected, acquired, transformed into a sparse domain and finally the sparse system matrix is reconstructed. Storing the system matrix in its sparse domain reduces the memory requirements. The reconstruction of the particle concentration may happen in the sparse domain as well [4]. The system functions that are the spatial distributions of one frequency component of the system matrix, can be sorted by their signal to noise ratio (SNR). Those system functions, whose SNR is above the noise level, are selected, transformed and used for further reconstruction. Applying a low SNR threshold of 10, the amount of selected system functions reduces to 3 %. For undersampled system functions the SNR can be estimated by the mixing order of the corresponding frequency [5]. The frequencies obtained in MPI can be displayed as a linear combination of the exciting frequencies. The sum of the coefficients of this linear combination determines the mixing order. A small mixing order corresponds to a high SNR. After selecting and transforming the system functions into a sparse domain, they are reconstructed and compressed. One of the main properties of the sparse domain is that many values are zero or near zero. Those values do not need to be stored as their impact on the reconstruction of the particle concentration is negligible. Discarding 90 % of the smallest values, there is no visible difference in the reconstruction. Applying both the compression and the SNR threshold, the system matrix shrinks to 0.03 % of its original size and can be stored in the main memory. Finally, undersampling cannot only be used to reduce the acquisition time of a system matrix, but also to improve the spatial resolution of an MPI measurement. The resolution depends on the discretisation of the FOV. Discretising a FOV with NxN pixels, the reconstruction results in an image of NxN pixels as well. When undersampled by a factor of 0.25, a FOV of 128x128 pixels can be fully acquired in the same time as a FOV of 64x64 pixels. As the size of the FOV is the same in both cases, undersampling the system matrix doubles the spatial resolution in two spatial directions.

[1] B. Gleich and J. Weizenecker. Tomographic Imaging Using the Nonlinear Response of Magnetic Particles. Nature, 435(7046):1214-7, 2005.

[2] E. J. Candès, J. Romberg and T. Tao. Robust Uncertainty Principles: Exact Signal Reconstruction from Highly Incomplete Frequency Information. IEEE Transactions on Information Theory, 52(2):489-509, 2006.

[3] T. Knopp and A. Weber. Sparse Reconstruction of the Magnetic Particle Imaging System Matrix. IEEE Transactions on Medical Imaging, 32(8):1473-1480, 2013.

[4] J. Lampe, C. Bassoy, J. Rahmer, J. Weizenecker, H. Voss, B. Gleich and J. Borgert. Fast Reconstruction in Magnetic Particle Imaging. Physics in Medicine and Biology, 57(4):1113-1134, 2012.

Corresponding Author: A. von Gladiß, vongladiss@gmx.de

[5] J. Rahmer, J. Weizenecker, B. Gleich and J. Borgert. Analysis of a 3-D System Function Measured for Magnetic Particle Imaging. IEEE Transactions on Medical Imaging, 31(6):1289-99, 2012.

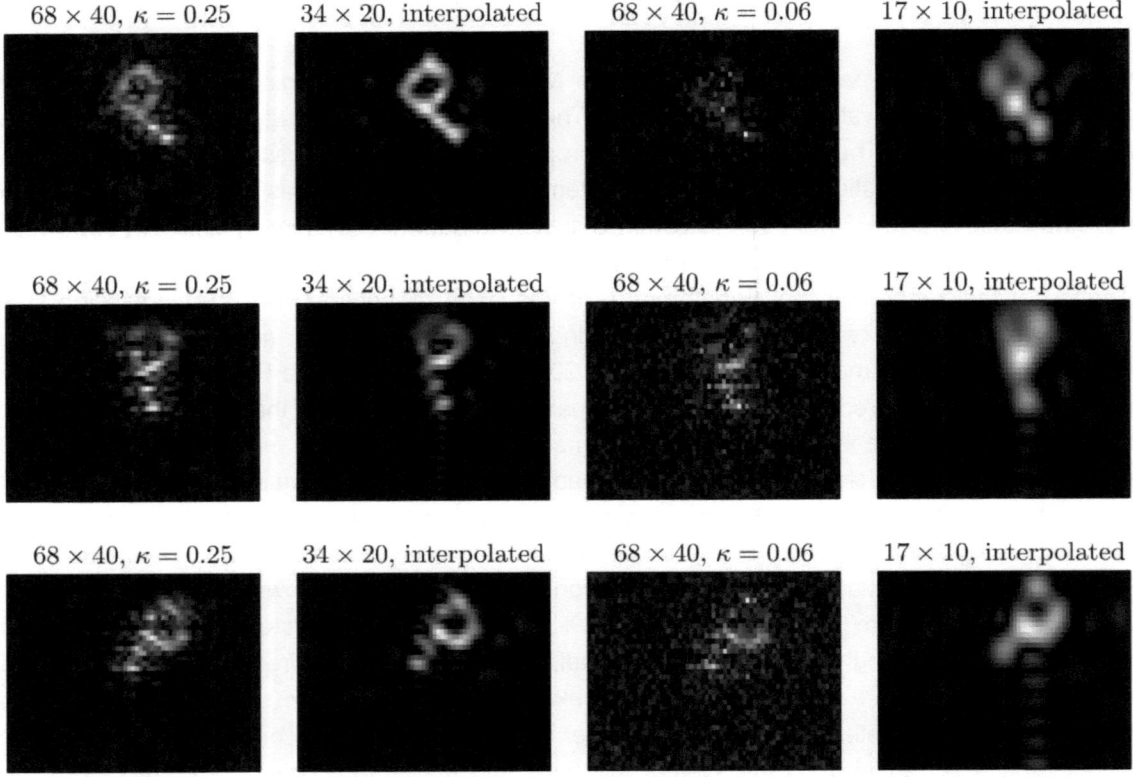

Reconstruction of a measured particle concentration with both an undersampled system matrix (first and third column) and a fully sampled system matrix with reduced discretisation of the FOV. The original FOV is discretised by 68x40 pixels and has been undersampled. In the second and fourth column it has been discretised by 34x20 and 17x10 pixels. As the undersampling factor κ indicates, the effort to sample the system matrix is the same for each pair of columns. After the reconstruction process, the images of the second and fourth columns have been interpolated in the Fourier domain to 68x40 pixels. Although the reconstruction of the second column has a stronger contrast and therefore seems to be better, spatial information is lost. The spaces between the single dots forming the phantom cannot be seen anymore (first row, second column). Reducing the discretisation even more, the phantom blurs and strong background artifacts appear. The original slight shape of the phantom blurs, but can still be recognized in the comparable reconstruction using a strongly undersampled system matrix.

Corresponding Author: A. von Gladiß, vongladiss@gmx.de

RECONSTRUCTION ENHANCEMENT BY USING FREQUENCY DOMAIN FILTERS

Alexander Weber[1], Jürgen Weizenecker[2], Jochen Franke[1], Ulrich Heinen[1], Michael Heidenreich[1], Wolfgang Ruhm[1], Thorsten Buzug[3]

[1]*Bruker Biospin MRI, Ettlingen, Germany*
[2]*University of Applied Siences, Karlsruhe, Germany*
[3]*Institute of Medical Engineering, University of Lübeck, Germany*

Magnetic particle imaging (MPI) is a new imaging modality which allows the detection of superparamagnetic iron oxide nanoparticles in vivo in three dimensions and in real time.

One approach to reconstruct the particle distribution is the system function method. In this method a linear system of equations has to be solved. Hereby the system matrix of the linear system describes the mapping between the MPI image and the signals induced in the receive coils.

Commonly the system matrix is determined by a calibration scan, where the system response of a small delta sample with the size of one voxel is measured at the various discretization positions of the field-of-view (FOV). Due to measurement-based determination the system matrix contains noise which is ideally caused by the thermal noise of the calibration sample, but more often is dominated by noise from components of the transmit/receive chain.

Because the system matrix exhibits a high condition number and both the system matrix and the measurement signal contain noise, the Tikhonov regularization is introduced to solve the linear system of equations.

Hereby a regularization parameter λ is used to prevent an overfitting of noise. Decreasing λ improves the resolution, but it also increases the noise floor and so the best trade-off between resolution and noise has to be found.

Furthermore, the linear system of equations is huge and so iterative algorithms are necessary to solve this problem. The optimum number of iterations depends on the noise floor of the system matrix, because increasing the iterations beyond a certain degree leads again to an overfitting.

To attenuate these effects of a noisy system matrix, a denoising method of the system matrix is proposed. To establish the denoising strategy, white noise is assumed [4] and because the system matrix components are well-compressible with the discrete Fourier transformation or the discrete Cosine transformation [2], frequency domain filters are chosen [1]. These filters exploit the fact that white noise is not compressible. Thus the true signal is located in a few coefficients after the transformation and the noise can be reduced by canceling coefficients which are smaller than a certain threshold parameter. This can be done by hard or soft thresholding. The threshold parameter is assessed to the variance of the noise, which can be estimated by the coefficients corresponding to high spatial frequencies of the system matrix components, because the true signal is expected to be located at small frequencies.

This method has been evaluated with data acquired at the preclinical demonstrator of Philips Research Hamburg. The measurement sequence has been a rotating P-Phantom which consists of twelve cylinders of length 1mm and diameter of 0.5mm filled with undiluted Resovist. The distance between these cylinders differs from 1.25 mm to 0.9 mm. The scanner setting has been carried out with a gradient of 5.5 T/m and a drive-field strength of 18mT. The FOV of 20.4 x 12.0 mm2 has been covered by a regular spatial grid of 68 x 40. To reconstruct the P-Phantom frequencies up to 1 MHz are used.

Corresponding Author: A. Weber, Alexander.Weber@bruker-biospin.de

Figure 1: (left) Reconstruction result with the original system matrix, regularization parameter $\lambda = 0.001$ and 7 iterations. (right) Reconstruction result with the denoised system matrix, regularization parameter $\lambda = 0.00005$ and 100 iterations. The denoised system matrix is obtained by the combination of the discrete Fourier Transformation and soft thresholding.

In figure 1 good reconstruction results with the original and the denoised system matrix are presented. The regularization parameter λ and the number of iterations are adapted by hand to achieve a good trade-off between resolution and the signal-to-noise ratio. It could be shown that after denoising the system matrix, the regularization parameter can be decreased and the number of iterations can be increased without an overfitting to noise. Because of this the resolution could be significant increased. There can be more cylinders be distinguished using the denoised system matrix in contrast to the original system matrix.

This method can be naturally combined with the sparse reconstruction method presented in [3]. Thereby the increase in reconstruction time because of the increase in the number of iterations can be at least equalized. Furthermore this method can be used to accelerate the calibration process of the system matrix because fewer averages are necessary to get a useful system matrix.

[1] A Buades et al, 2005, A Review of Image Denoising Algorithms, with a New One, Multiscale Model. Simul., 4, 490-530

[2] T Knopp and A Weber 2013, Sparse Reconstruction of the magnetic particle imaging system matrix, IEEE Trans Med Imaging, 32, 1473-80

[3] J Lampe et al, 2012, Fast Reconstruction in Magnetic Particle Imaging, Medical Physics, 37, 485-491

[4] J Weizenecker et al, 2007, A simulation study on the resolution and sensitivity of magnetic particle imaging, Physics in Medicine and Biology, 53, 6363-6374

Corresponding Author: A. Weber, Alexander.Weber@bruker-biospin.de

A PHENOMENOLOGICAL DESCRIPTION OF THE MPS-SIGNAL USING A MODEL FOR THE FIELD DEPENDENCE OF THE EFFECTIVE RELAXATION TIME

Daniel Schmidt[1], Florian Palmetshofer[1], David Heinke[2], Uwe Steinhoff[1], Frank Ludwig[3]

[1]*Physikalisch-Technische Bundesanstalt, Berlin, Germany*
[2]*nanoPET Pharma GmbH, Berlin, Germany*
[3]*Institute of Electrical Measurement and Fundamental Electrical Engineering, Braunschweig, Germany*

In the last years, Magnetic Particle Spectroscopy (MPS) has become one of the most powerful tools to characterize magnetic nanoparticles (MNP) for MPI. For a detailed understanding of MNP dynamics a consistent simulation of the MPS signal is of considerable interest.

One approach is to model single particle dynamics based on the Gilbert-Landau-Lifschitz equation and then integrate the results over a wide range of parameters in order to represent a realistic MNP ensemble. However, the real distribution of parameters like anisotropy constant, effective magnetic diameter or moment per particle can only be estimated from measurements and forms a prominent source of uncertainty in the results. Mathematical models for the dynamic behavior of an MNP ensemble do exist only for special cases, eg. for small excitation fields or for limited field directions.

Our goal is to establish a simple model of MNP dynamics which is only based on physical quantities directly accessible by measurements. This model incorporates the data from $M(H)$ measurements and the relaxation time τ at a magnetic field $H=0$ as it is detected by magnetorelaxometry (MRX). The behavior of τ at larger drive field amplitudes is represented by a phenomenological expression which can be parameterized:

$$\tau(H) = \tau(H=0)/(1+a\cdot H^b). \quad (1)$$

We start from the well known dynamic behavior of the magnetic moment of an ensemble of MNP near $H=0$:

$$m(t) = \chi \cdot V \cdot H - \tau \cdot (dm/dt). \quad (2)$$

This first order linear differential equation based on the magnetic moment m of a particle sample and the relaxation time τ is modeled and eventually solved. Here, χ represents the total magnetic susceptibility of the sample and V is the sample volume.

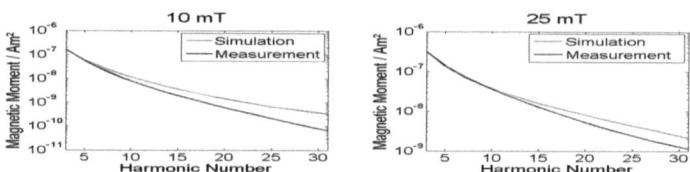

Fig 1. Comparison of MPS measurements and simulation results for different field strengths.

Implementing in a further modeling step a magnetic field dependent effective relaxation time $\tau(H)$ and susceptibility $\chi(H)$ leads to a coupled system of differential equations. In order to solve that system, we discretize the problem into small steps with fixed but updated values for $\tau(H)$ and $\chi(H)$ and derive a numerical solution for the dynamic behavior. The values for $\chi(H)$ are obtained from quasistatic $M(H)$ measurements.

Corresponding Author: D. Schmidt, daniel.schmidt@ptb.de

The relaxation time at zero field detected by MRX resulted in a boundary condition for the analytical expression of τ(H). To find the parameters a and b of τ(H), we compared simulated to measured MPS spectra and minimized the difference by a correlation analysis. It is shown for different real particle systems, that this method is suitable to describe the MPS spectra at 10 mT and 25 mT with MNP specific fit parameters a and b obtaining a correlation of at least $R^2=0.99$ (see fig. 1). Therefore the method might be used to investigate and characterize dynamic behavior of MNP based only on directly measurable parameters.

Acknowledgements: This work was supported by the German Federal Ministry of Economics and Technology grant No. KF2303711UW2, KF3061201UW2 and KF2725002UW2.

Corresponding Author: D. Schmidt, daniel.schmidt@ptb.de

DEBYE-BASED FREQUENCY-DOMAIN MAGNETIZATION MODEL FOR MAGNETIC NANOPARTICLES AND ITS APPLICATION TO VISCOSITY-DEPENDENT MPS MEASUREMENTS

Thilo Wawrzik, Meinhard Schilling, Frank Ludwig

Institut fuer Elektrische Messtechnik und Grundlagen der Elektrotechnik, Technische Universität Braunschweig, Germany

Theoretical descriptions and numerical simulations in the context of magnetic particle imaging (MPI) and magnetic particle spectroscopy (MPS) are historically based on the Langevin function of superparamagnetism. Since the static nature of that equation does not suffice to cover the magnetization dynamics involved in MPI signal generation, the Langevin function is usually extended via a frequency-dependent term based on the Debye model, which has been successfully employed in the field of ac susceptibility measurements. As it turns out, the standard Debye model was derived to cover the frequency dependence of the base frequency only (ac susceptibility uses a lock-in detection principle to obtain magnitude and phase of the detection signal). However, the interest in higher harmonics for MPI sets the need to include these harmonics into the model formalism. From MPS evaluation it is well-known that both magnitude and phase of the particle signal depend on the excitation frequency as well as on the harmonic index in the observed spectrum.

We derived a simple equation, where each harmonic is multiplied with a complex-valued weighting factor, using familiar semantics of the χ' and χ'' notation. The resulting spectrum is represented as a sum of weighted harmonics. Since the description of the spectrum and the frequency-dependent modification are formulated in frequency space, the evaluation of the model is computationally cheap and allows one to apply the model to complex scenarios, such as non-linear optimization, i.e., fitting the model to a measured particle spectrum.

It is shown, that in the context of viscosity-dependent MPS spectra, the model proofs to be applicable for estimating the viscosity of the measured particle system. While viscosity is the parameter of choice for an experimental validation, the ultimate goal is the more general use of the model for determining the hydrodynamic volume or the binding state of the particles.

Acknowledgement: This work was supported by the German Federal Ministry of Economics and Technology under grant No. FKZ KF3061201UW2.

Session 4

MPI Theory, Relaxometry, Magnetometry

Chairs: J. Weaver, L. Trahms

SIMULTANEOUS RECONSTRUCTION AND RESOLUTION ENHANCEMENT FOR MAGNETIC PARTICLE IMAGING

Osama A. Omer[1,2], Hanne Wojtczyk[1], Thorsten M. Buzug[1]

[1]*Institute of Medical Engineering, University of Lübeck, Germany*
[2]*Electrical Engineering Department, Aswan University, Egypt*

An essential parameter of magnetic particle imaging (MPI) is the spatial resolution [1,2]. The spatial resolution of MPI depends, among other things, on the particles' diameter and the sampling frequency. The spatial resolution increases when increasing the particle diameter. However, large particles suffer from relaxation effects and are not preferred in some applications. On the other hand, spatial resolution increases with the sampling frequency, which in turn increases the number of sampling points. As an alternative solution for resolution enhancement, super-resolution (SR) [3] can be beneficial in improving the image quality of many medical imaging systems without the need for significant hardware alteration. In this paper, we propose to use small particle diameter and low sampling frequency to reconstruct multiple magnetic particle images with low-resolution (LR) and apply a resolution enhancement technique to reconstruct a higher resolution magnetic particle image. Unlike the conventional SR techniques, we propose to reconstruct a high-resolution (HR) image from the measured LR signals instead of reconstructing LR images and then post-process these images to get a higher resolution image. Simulation results show that using simultaneous reconstruction and resolution enhancement results in sharper images and more robust against noise than using SR as a post process.

Rather than performing resolution enhancement in two steps, HR MPI reconstruction problem can be described as to minimize

$$J(\underline{X}) = \sum_{k=1}^{N} \left[\left\| \mathbf{GDBW}_k \underline{X} - \underline{U}_k \right\|_2^2 \right] + \lambda \left\| \mathbf{H} \underline{X} \right\|_2^2 \tag{1}$$

where **G** is the system matrix, $\underline{U}_k$ is the kth measured signal, $\mathbf{W}_k$ is the geometric motion operator between the HR image $\underline{X}$ and the kth LR concentration, **B** is the blurring operator, λ is the regularization parameter, **D** is the down-sampling operator and **H** is a high-pass filter operator.

Results and discussion of a simulation study
Figure 1b-d shows the reconstruction results in case of using sampling frequency (Fs) of 2 MHz and particle diameter (D) of 50 nm. The reconstructed LR image is shown in Fig. 1b. Figure 1c shows the super resolved reconstructed MPI by using SR as a post-process by combining 4 LR images. The reconstructed HR MPI image is shown in Fig. 1d. Further results for other parameter combinations are depicted in Figs. 1e-1m. From these images, we can see that the super resolved MPI image is blurred compared to the reconstructed HR MPI, that is because of the double regularization in the two cascaded stages, reconstruction and super-resolution.

Acknowledgments
This work is funded in part by the Egyptian Ministry of High Education and DAAD through the GERSS program. Also, the authors gratefully acknowledge the financial support of the German Federal Ministry of Education and Research (BMBF) under grant number 13N11090 and of the European Union and the State Schleswig-Holstein (Programme for the Future – Economy) under grant number 122-10-004.

Corresponding Author: O. Omer, omer.osama@gmail.com

[1] B. Gleich and J. Weizenecker, "Tomographic imaging using the nonlinear response of magnetic particles," Nature, vol. 435, pp. 1214–1217, 2005.

[2] B. Gleich, J. Weizenecker, and J. Borgert, "Experimental results on fast 2D-encoded magnetic particle imaging," Physics in Medicine and Biology, vol. 53, pp. N81–N84, 2008.

[3] P. Milanfar, "Super-Resolution Imaging," CRC Press, September 2010.

[4] T. Knopp, T. F. Sattel, S. Biederer, J. Rahmer, J. Weizenecker, B. Gleich, J. Borgert, and T. M. Buzug, "Model-based reconstruction for magnetic particle imaging," IEEE Trans. Med. Imaging, vol. 29, no. 1, pp. 12–18, 2010.

[5] H. Greenspan, "Super-Resolution in Medical Imaging," The Computer Journal, vol. 52, No. 1, pp. 43-63, 2009.

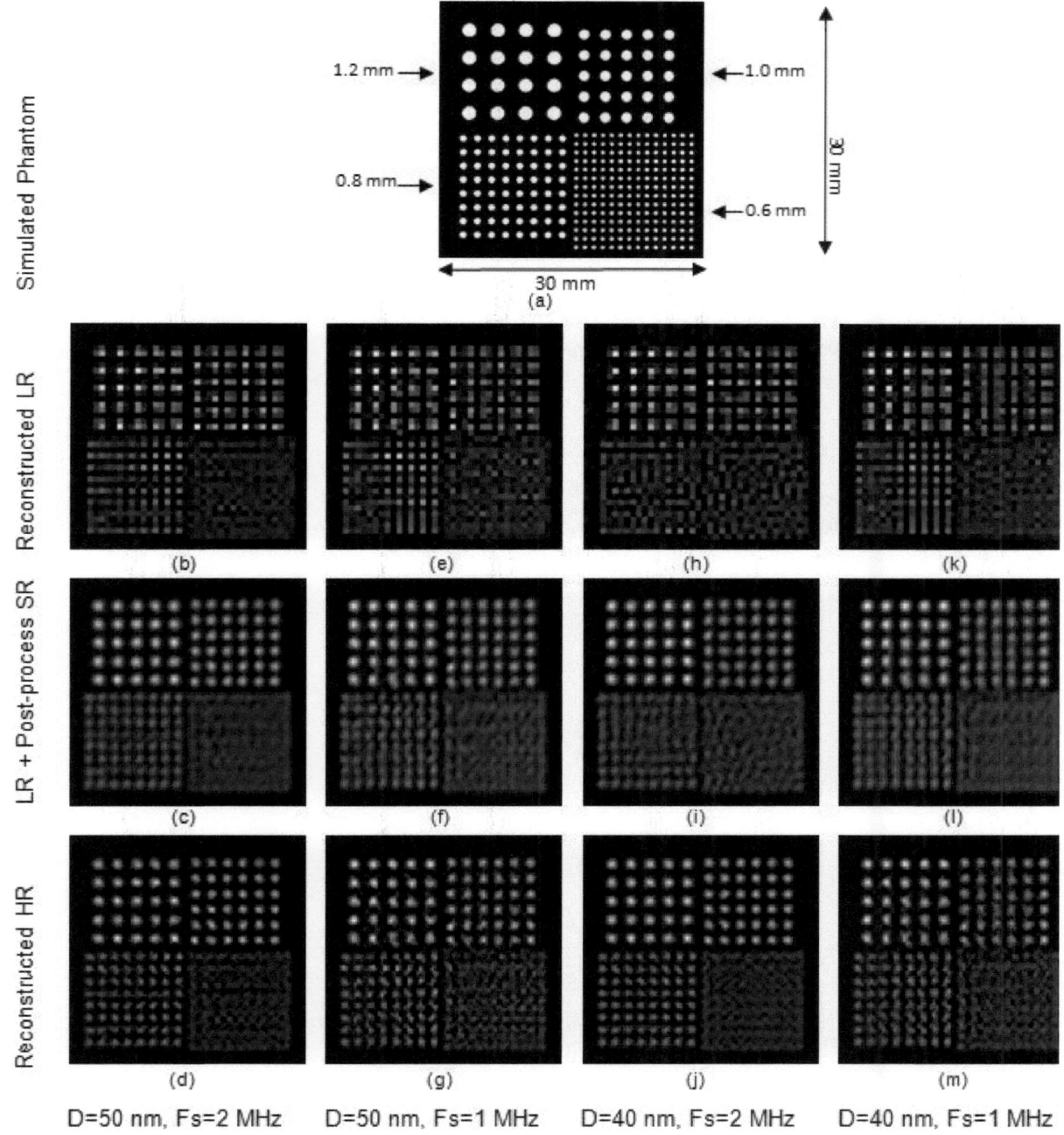

Figure 1, reconstructed images with different methods

Corresponding Author: O. Omer, omer.osama@gmail.com

FIELD DEPENDENT CHARACTERISTIC TIMESCALES FOR MAGNETIC NANOPARTICLE ROTATIONS

Daniel B. Reeves[1], John B. Weaver[2]

[1]Dept. of Physics and Astronomy, Dartmouth College, Hanover, USA
[2]Dept. of Radiology, Geisel School of Medicine, Hanover, USA

The physics of magnetic nanoparticles in an applied field depends strongly on the type and strength of the field applied. There are two relaxation mechanisms (internal—Néel and external—Brown) and both are useful for different purposes in medical and biosensing technologies. The two mechanisms are often differentiated by their relaxation times. Yet, these times are defined by the relaxation back to equilibrium, and when particles are driven with high fields, they are not necessarily at equilibrium at all. Instead, it makes sense to examine the different "characteristic timescales" that arise due to varying applied fields. Several approximations have been made previously, and we summarize the possible approaches. We show how the large field relaxation time can be derived from a Langevin equation approach, and lastly compare all the models to simulated data from numerically integrated stochastic differential equations.

Corresponding Author: D. B. Reeves, dbr@dartmouth.edu

DEPENDENCE OF BROWNIAN AND NÉEL RELAXATION TIMES ON MAGNETIC FIELD STRENGTH

Robert J. Deissler

Case Western Reserve University, Cleveland, USA

Purpose: In Magnetic Particle Imaging (MPI) and Magnetic Particle Spectroscopy (MPS) the relaxation time of the magnetization in response to externally applied magnetic fields is determined by the Brownian and Néel relaxation mechanisms. Here we investigate the dependence of the relaxation times on the magnetic field strength and the implications for MPI and MPS.

Methods: The Fokker-Planck equation with Brownian relaxation and the Fokker-Planck equation with Néel relaxation are solved numerically for a time-varying externally applied magnetic field, including a step-function, a sinusoidally varying, and a linearly ramped magnetic field. For magnetic fields that are applied as a step function, an eigenvalue approach is used to directly calculate both the Brownian and Néel relaxation times for a range of magnetic field strengths. For Néel relaxation, the eigenvalue calculations are compared to Brown's high-barrier approximation formula.

Results: The relaxation times due to the Brownian or Néel mechanisms depend on the magnitude of the applied magnetic field. In particular, the Néel relaxation time is sensitive to the magnetic field strength, and varies by many orders of magnitude for nanoparticle properties and magnetic field strengths relevant for MPI and MPS. Therefore, the well-known zero-field relaxation times underestimate the actual relaxation times and, in particular, can underestimate the Néel relaxation time by many orders of magnitude. When only Néel relaxation is present -- if the particles are embedded in a solid for instance -- we found that there can be a strong magnetization response to a sinusoidal driving field, even if the period is much less than the zero-field relaxation time. For a ferrofluid in which both Brownian and Néel relaxation are present, only one relaxation mechanism may dominate depending on the magnetic field strength, the driving frequency (or ramp time), and the phase of the magnetization relative to the applied magnetic field.

Conclusions: A simple treatment of Néel relaxation using the common zero-field relaxation time overestimates the relaxation time of the magnetization in situations relevant for MPI and MPS. For sinusoidally driven (or ramped) systems, whether or not a particular relaxation mechanism dominates or is even relevant depends on the magnetic field strength, the frequency (or ramp time), and the phase of the magnetization relative to the applied magnetic field.

Corresponding Author: R. Deissler, rjd42@case.edu

HANDHELD DIFFERENTIAL MAGNETOMETRY WITH A SPLIT COIL GEOMETRY

Sebastiaan Waanders, Tasio Oderkerk, Martijn Visscher, Erik Krooshoop, Bennie ten Haken

MIRA Institute for Biomedical Technology and Technical Medicine, University of Twente
Enschede, The Netherlands

Differential magnetometry allows for fast, accurate measurement of small amounts of SPIO nanoparticles in biological tissue. For handheld applications, i.e. for use in intra-operative settings, spatial and temporal resolution need to be high, using simple, robust hardware. This poses a challenge for conventional magnetometer design, as sensing depth and accuracy are ultimately limited by the excitation and detection coil diameter. In this paper, we describe a split coil geometry, in which we separate the (large) excitation coil from the small detection coil. This allows for significantly increased depth sensitivity, due to the larger excitation coil diameter, which is placed under the subject of interest. This is especially relevant for intra-operative procedures, for example during magnetic sentinel lymph node mapping[1].

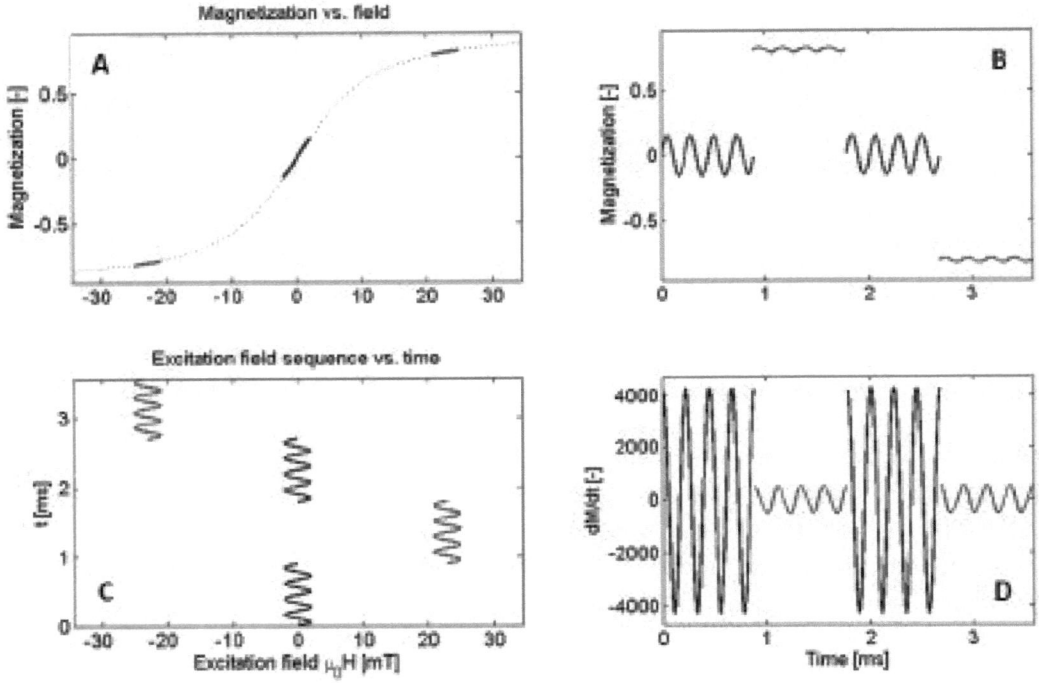

Figure 1: Schematic representation of the DiffMag concept. SPIO nanoparticles (A) are exposed to a constant AC field, periodically modulated by quasi-static offset fields, which drive the particles towards saturation (B). This results in a modulation of the particle's magnetization (C), which results in a changing induced voltage in the detection coil (D).

By using the DiffMag protocol (illustrated in Figure 1), which is discrete in time by alternating periods of AC excitation (with frequencies up to 10 kHz) with periods in which an offset field is added, we are able to separate the signal coming from the changing mutual inductance from the SPIO nanoparticle signal. This allows us to accurately and rapidly locate the SPIO nanoparticles, for example during a magnetic sentinel node biopsy. This is impossible in conventional magnetometry, as the rapidly varying mutual inductance between excitation- and detection coils during probe movement quickly obfuscates any signal coming from the SPIO nanoparticles.

Corresponding Author: S. Waanders, s.waanders@utwente.nl

The concept of handheld differential magnetometry is currently being verified in an ex vivo trial in which, after a subareolar injection of Resovist®, the complete breast volume and lymphatic basin are excised. Afterwards, a magnetic sentinel node biopsy is performed on the tissue to assess the viability of this technique and compare it to existing magnetic and radioactive methods. Phantom experiments indicate a detection limit of ~1µg, and we are exploring additional ways of improving this, for example by cooling the detection coil using a state-of-the-art miniature cryocooler[2].

Together with two local hospitals and a broad spectrum of industry partners ranging from industrial designers to health & safety professionals, we are currently evaluating the viability of this clinical prototype for an intraoperative setting. CE marking of the probe and complementary hardware is planned for next year, with in vivo clinical evaluation planned for 2015.

In addition to the handheld magnetometer system, we construct a standalone magnetometer similar to an MPI spectrometer[3] or relaxometer[4], which is able to rapidly quantify the amount of nanoparticles present in, for example, an excised lymph node or tumor volume. To quantitatively assess the performance of various SPIO nanoparticles in different media, the rapid DiffMag protocol allows us to follow biological processes like protein adhesion to the nanoparticles[5] in real time by monitoring their (Brownian) relaxation time constants (derived from the differential magnetization curve, dM/dH), which is critical for predicting tracer behavior in complex body fluids. The relatively low excitation frequency enables us to trace these phenomena by virtue of the device's high sensitivity for changes in particle diameter due to the changing Brownian time constants. The DiffMag quantitative magnetometer operates at low power and small magnetic field strengths of around 10-25mT, without the need for magnetic shielding, making it very suitable for clinical applications.

[1] Ahmed, M., & Douek, M. (2013). The role of magnetic nanoparticles in the localization and treatment of breast cancer. BioMed research international, 2013, 281230. doi:10.1155/2013/281230

[2] Brake, H. J. M. ter, Burger, J. F., Holland, H. J., Derking, J. H., Rogalla, H., & Lerou, P. P. P. (2008). Micromachined cryogenic coolers for cooling low-temperature detectors and electronics. 2008 IEEE Sensors. doi:10.1109/ICSENS.2008.4716696

[3] Biederer, S., Sattel, T., Knopp, T., Gleich, B., Weizenecker, J., Borgert, J., & Buzug, T. M. (2009). A Spectrometer for Magnetic Particle Imaging. In IFMBE Proceedings, Volume 22 (pp. 2313–2316). doi:10.1007/978-3-540-89208-3_555

[4] Goodwill, P. W., Tamrazian, A., Croft, L. R., Lu, C. D., Johnson, E. M., Pidaparthi, R., ... Conolly, S. M. (2011). Ferrohydrodynamic relaxometry for magnetic particle imaging. Applied Physics Letters, 98(26), 262502. doi:10.1063/1.3604009

[5] Jedlovszky-Hajdú, A., Bombelli, F. B., Monopoli, M. P., Tombácz, E., & Dawson, K. a. (2012). Surface coatings shape the protein corona of SPIONs with relevance to their application in vivo. Langmuir : the ACS journal of surfaces and colloids, 28, 14983–91. doi:10.1021/la302446h

Corresponding Author: S. Waanders, s.waanders@utwente.nl

Session 5

Magnetic Nanoparticles & Tracer Materials

Chairs: G. Schuetz, M. Taupitz

Keynote

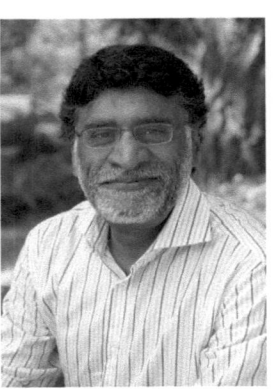

Prof. Kannan Krishnan

Materials Science & Engineering, University of Washington, USA

Optimized tracers for MPI: Progress and Challenges

DYNAMIC MAGNETIC BEHAVIOUR OF DDM128 IN AGAROSE GEL, GELATINE AND SUGAR MATRIX

Dietmar Eberbeck, Lutz Trahms

Physikalisch-Technische Bundesanstalt, Berlin, Germany

The efficiency of the MPI strongly depends on the structure of the applied magnetic nanoparticles (MNP) such as magnetic moment and magnetic anisotropy. However, in case of larger MNP a strong magnetic dipole-dipole interaction (DDI) can occur determined by the particle correlation within the given matrix (tissue, gels) [1]. Thus, DDI co-determines significantly the magnetic behaviour.

We investigated MNP of different fractions of DDM128, obtained by static magnetic fractionation, where we focus on the fractions E500 with a mean effective magnetic diameter of d_V=20 nm and E12 with d_V=29 nm. Interestingly, the initial magnetic bimodality of DDM128 persists after fractionation. Thus, we conclude that the fractionated MNP have a multicore structure with an inhomogeneous magnetisation.

MNP of DDM128, E500 and E12 were embedded in a sugar matrix, in gelatine and agarose gel. We found that there is a significant difference between the corresponding Magnetic Particle Spectroscopy (MPS) data, M(H) curves and Magnetorelaxometry (MRX) data of MNP immobilised in sugar matrix on the one hand and in the gel matrices on the other hand. While this difference in M(H)-data amounts to about 15% for DDM128 and E500 it reaches 60% in case of E12. This may be attributed to the larger magnetic moments (stronger interaction). This is also reflected by MRX and MPS measurements: The amplitude spectra of MPS, $A(k)$ (k-order of the harmonics), and the phase curves $\phi(k)$ of E500 samples (all immobilisations) and of E12 in sugar matrix are qualitatively similar. In contrast, E12 in gelatine and agarose shows a steeper decay in A_k. The phase behaviour ϕ_k of E12 in agarose is very similar to that of E12 in sugar matrix but ϕ_k of E12 in gelatine strongly differs from that of the other samples.

Using different sensitive magnetic measurement techniques, we found evidence of a complex particle structure in preparations of multicore MNP and we could discriminate between 3 obviously qualitatively different MNP superstructures in different matrices. Obviously, these different structures affect the MPS-behaviour via the dipole-dipole-interaction.

Corresponding Author: D. Eberbeck, dietmar.eberbeck@ptb.de

DEPENDENCE OF TEMPERATURE PROBING ON TAYLOR'S EXPANSION OF LANGEVIN FUNCTION USING MAGNETIC NANOPARTICLES IN DC FIELD

Ling Jiang, Wenzhong Liu, Jing Zhong, Pu Zhang

School of Automation, Huazhong University of Science and Technology, Wuhan, China

Temperature probing using magnetic nanoparticles is a promising technique, which has potential of probing temperature *in vivo* noninvasively [1-5]. Magnetization curve of magnetic nanoparticles is sensitive to temperature, which can be described by Langevin function. In our recent paper, temperature probing using magnetic nanoparticles was achieved by using Taylor's expansion of Langevin function [4, 5]. According to the described model, the temperature estimation error resource dates from truncation error of Taylor's expansion, solving error of system function, and magnetization measurement noise. However, none of the impact factors has been studied. In this paper, we study the dependence of temperature probing on Taylor's expansion order of Langevin function by simulation. Temperature probing was achieved by using magnetization curves and matrix equation solving. Fig. 1 shows the temperature probing errors in different Taylor's expansion orders. It indicates that the absolute error of temperature probing firstly decreases and then increases with an increase in expansion order. Moreover, the inset shows that the standard deviation increases as an increase in expansion order. The explanation is that, with the same SNR of magnetization measurement, the error of temperature probing, mainly, dates from the truncation error of Taylor's expansion firstly and then dates from solving error of system function. As the order of Taylor's expansion increases, the truncation error decreases while the solving error of system function increases. Herein, the solving error of system function is determined by magnetization measurement noise and matrix condition number. The increasing of matrix condition number with expansion order (seen in the inset) enlarges the impact of magnetization measurement noise. Therefore, the standard deviation of temperature probing errors monotonically increases.

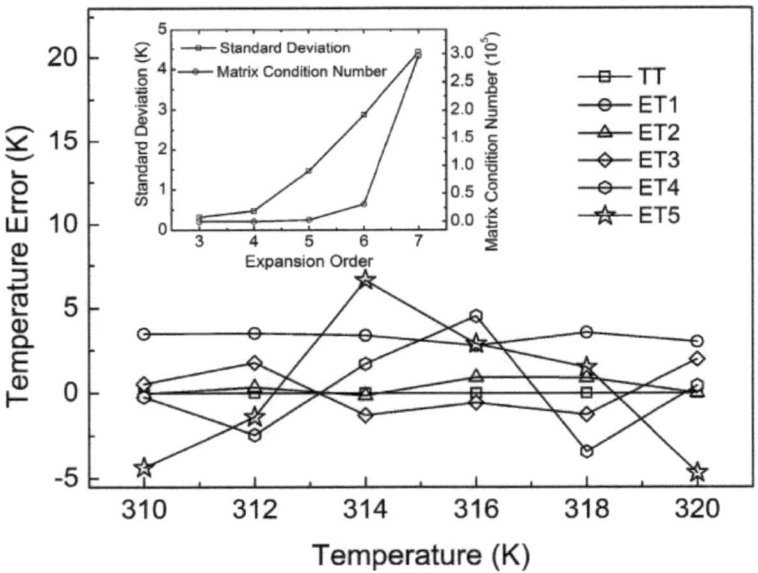

Fig. 1. Temperature probing error in different expansion orders of Langevin function. ET1-ET5 represent the temperature probing errors in 3rd, 4th, 5th, 6th, and 7th order of Taylor's expansion. The inset shows the standard deviation of estimated errors in different expansion orders. The applied magnetic fields are from -200 Gauss to 200 Gauss with a step of 10 Gauss. And the effective magnetic moment is 1×10^{-19} emu.

Corresponding Author: W. Liu, lwz7410@hust.edu.cn

[1] G. Kucsko, P. C. Maurer, N. Y. Yao, M. Kubo, H. J. Noh, P. K. Lo, H. Park, and M. D. Lukin, Nanometre-scale thermometry in a living cell, *Nature*, **500,** 54 (2013).

[2] Gigi Galiana, Rosa T. Branca, Elizabeth R. Jenista, Warren S. Warren, Accurate Temperature Imaging Based on Intermolecular Coherences in Magnetic Resonance, *Science*, **322,** 421 (2008).

[3] John B. Weaver, Adam M. Rauwerdink and Eric W. Hansen, Magnetic nanoparticle temperature estimation, *Medical Physics*, **36,** 1822 (2009).

[4] Jing Zhong, Wenzhong Liu, Zhongzhou Du, Paulo césar de Morais, Qing Xiang and Qingguo Xie, A noninvasive, remote and precise method for temperature and concentration estimation using magnetic nanoparticles, *Nanotechnology*, **23,** 075703 (2012).

[5] Yin Li, Wenzhong Liu and Jing Zhong, Comparison of noninvasive and remote temperature estimation employing magnetic nanoparticles in DC and AC applied fields, *Proceedings of I2MTC*, Graz, Austria, 2012, 2738-2741.

Corresponding Author: W. Liu, lwz7410@hust.edu.cn

SYNTHETIC APPROACHES FOR IRON OXIDE NANOPARTICLES SUITABLE AS TRACER FOR MAGNETIC PARTICLE IMAGING

Andreas Ide, Farnoosh Roohi, Hubertus Pietsch, Gunnar Schuetz

MR & CT Contrast Media Research, BayerHealthcare, Berlin, Germany

Magnetic Particle Imaging (MPI) is a novel tomographic imaging modality currently under development. MPI visualizes magnetic nanoparticles quantitatively at a high temporal and spatial resolution. These three features bear the potential for MPI to become a competitive diagnostic imaging modality. After intravenous injection of magnetic nanoparticles their distribution can be followed by a temporal resolution of up to 46 frames per second. Moving organs like the heart as well as catheter based interventional procedures may thus be followed in real-time. So that nanoparticles are able to fully exploit the potentials of MPI they must have particular magnetic properties. Those are very important, to enable a synergistic effect with the technical features of the MPI instruments. An improved tracer performance can spare extensive technical specifications of the instruments whereas a poor tracer performance raises the need for a more sophisticated instrumentation.

In order to be innovative in diagnostic imaging MPI has to provide additional diagnostic values, which cannot be obtained by improving established diagnostic imaging modalities. Currently, no tracer material is available that has magnetic properties being sufficient for the generation of such diagnostic value. An ideal tracer consists of iron oxide nanoparticles that ought to be magnetic and proofed to be biocompatible. A large number of super-paramagnetic iron oxide nanoparticles have been synthesized and used in animal studies as well as in human diagnostic procedures for magnetic resonance imaging over the last decades. Unfortunately, none of the reported SPIO formulations exhibit the desired magnetic properties for their use as MPI tracer. Resovist is the only SPIO formulation approved for clinical use as MR contrast agent that also generates a signal in MPI. Although it is unlikely that the MPI signal obtained with Resovist is sufficient for a competitive use in diagnostic imaging, it is regarded as gold standard for novel MPI tracer approaches. In order to exploit the full potential of MPI we investigated synthetic approaches to generate suitable iron oxide nanoparticles.

During the synthesis of iron oxide nanoparticles a number of chemical and physical properties were addressed in a single step. Especially the high magnetic dipole moment that gives rise to high sensitivity and spatial resolution was coded, not only in the crystal phase and size, but also in the inner nanoparticle structure. These parameters together define the magnetic anisotropy and saturation magnetization which are the key parameters. Therefore a well-tailored synthesis protocol is crucial for the final tracer performance. We synthesized MPI tracer particles exhibiting a magnetic dipole moment comparable to that of Resovist using different synthetic routes and thus gained substantial experience in fine-tuning of the desired magnetic properties. The precise understanding of the influence of various reaction parameters on the magnetic dipole moment of the resulting particles now allows directed synthesis approaches to generate novel MPI tracer.

Acknowledgments

The work is funded by the German Federal Ministry of Education and Research (BMBF), grant FKZ 13N11087.

Corresponding Author: A. Ide, Andreas.ide@bayer.com

PERPENDICULAR MAGNETIC PARTICLE IMAGING, PMPI

John B. Weaver

Department of Radiology, Dartmouth-Hitchcock Medical Center and Dartmouth College, One Medical Center Drive, Lebanon, US

The magnetization of an ensemble of magnetic nanoparticles in an alternating magnetic field flips with the field. Normally the magnetization perpendicular to the axis of the alternating field is zero because the forces on the nanoparticles are symmetric so there is no preferred direction. However, a relatively small static field can be applied perpendicular to the alternating field to produce a small pulse of magnetization as the alternating field passes through zero. The static field oriented perpendicular to the alternating field will disrupt the symmetry of the magnetizations as they pass through the plane perpendicular to the alternating field inducing a magnetization pulse perpendicular to the drive field. The perpendicular pickup coil is geometrically decoupled from the alternating drive field and static fields induce no current so the feedthrough can be very small enabling very high sensitivity to the magnetization pulse. If the alternating drive field is very large and the perpendicular field is relatively small, the perpendicular magnetization is a very short pulse. The pulse occurs when the alternating field passes through zero or slightly after if the relaxation is significant. Localization along any direction can be achieved by imposing a static gradient field in that direction; the field is in the direction of the alternating field but the gradient in that field can be any direction. The gradient makes the total field pass through zero at different times for each position along the gradient. Thus the nanoparticles from each position along the gradient produces signal at different times during the cycle of the alternating field allowing a one-dimensional projection to be produced. Rotating the gradient in three-dimensions and taking projections along each rotated direction allows a three-dimensional image to be produced. The process of imaging magnetic nanoparticles using the perpendicular field is termed pMPI.

We simulated pMPI for fast relaxation using the Langevin equation, equilibrium approximation to the magnetization. It is well known that a single signal peak from each position is generated in conventional MPI but the magnetization is a pulse in pMPI so the signal is a bipolar shape. The signal from 100nm nanoparticles provides reasonable resolution with 80mT alternating field and 75mT/m gradients. By varying the spatial resolution and calculating the conditioning allowed, pMPI can be compared to MPI. These very preliminary results indicate that the optimum conditioning achieved for pMPI required roughly three times the gradient in the MPI geometry. However, these preliminary results require more study.

Several permutations are possible. For example, three-dimensional imaging could be achieved using a modified MRI system where the main field is replaced by an alternating field and a static field coil / pickup coil combination were added. It is also feasible to image magnetic nanoparticles at much higher concentrations in an MRI system if the main field is used as the perpendicular static field and an alternating field is added perpendicular to the main field.

Corresponding Author: J. B. Weaver, john.b.weaver@dartmouth.edu

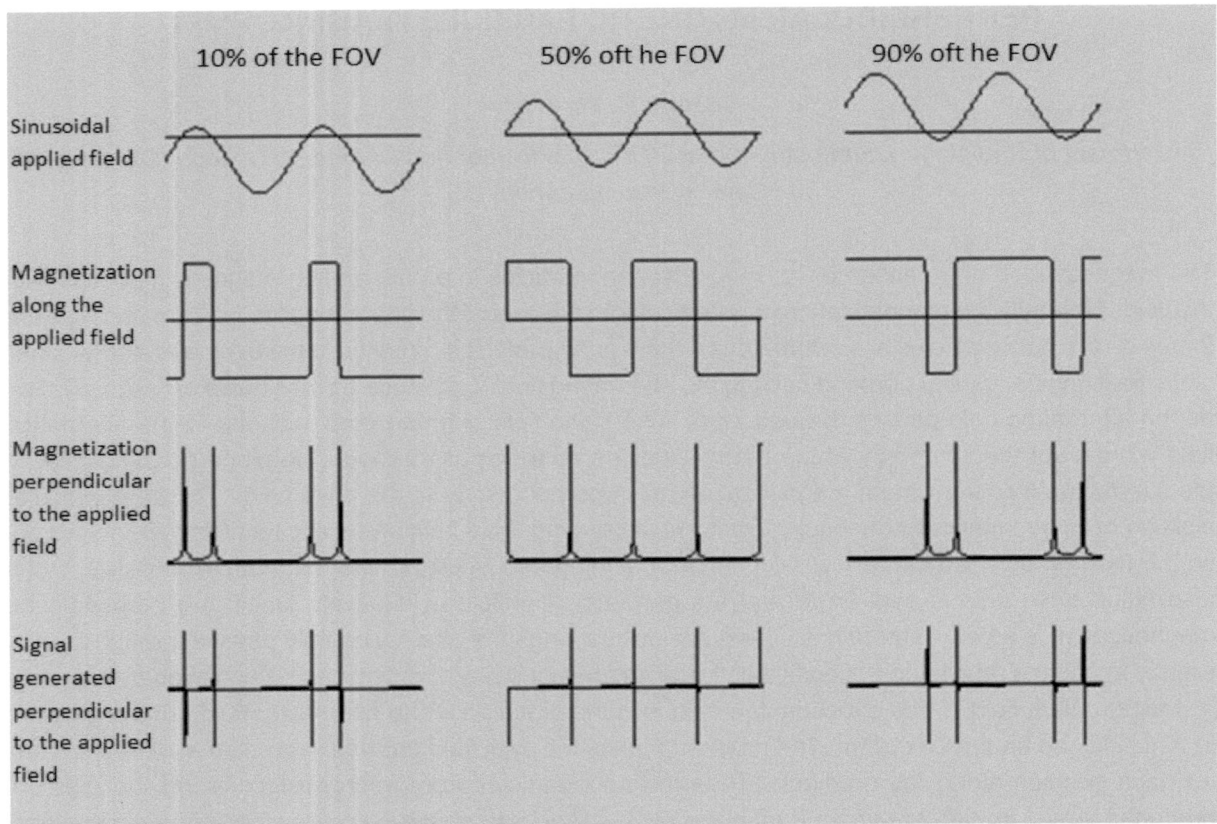

Fig. 1: A simulation assuming fast relaxation approximated by the Langevin function of the applied field. The sinusoidal applied field is 80 mT in amplitude; the gradient is 75 mT across the field of view (FOV); the nanoparticles are 100nm in diameter. Each column of the figure shows the following for three points across the FOV: the applied field (top), the magnetization in the direction oft he applied field (second row), the magnetization in the direction perpendicular tot he applied field (third row), and the detected signal from the magnetization in the perpendicular direction (last row). The first and third columns are 10% of the FOV from the edges oft he FOV and the second column is in the middle oft he FOV. The timing oft he signal generated allows the location of the nanoparticles producing the signal to be estimated.

Corresponding Author: J. B. Weaver, john.b.weaver@dartmouth.edu

Session 6

Magnetic Nanoparticles & Tracer Materials II

Chairs: K. Krishnan, J. Niehaus

OPTIMIZED MPI TRACERS PERFORM WELL OVER A RANGE OF EXCITATION FIELD CONDITIONS

R. Matthew Ferguson[1], Scott J. Kemp[1], Amit P. Khandhar[2], Kannan M. Krishnan[2]

[1]Lodespin Labs, Washington, USA
[2]Materials Science & Engineering, University of Washington, USA

Excitation fields of ~20 mT amplitude and 25 kHz are most common in the MPI literature up to the present time. However, to avoid peripheral nerve stimulation, future scanners may be designed with reduced excitation field amplitudes. Higher frequencies may also be utilized to recover signal to noise ratio (SNR) that is lost as a result of lower excitation field amplitudes. Modifying the excitation field will also affect the MPI tracer magnetic response and potentially affect the spatial resolution and sensitivity achievable in MPI. It is therefore necessary to understand how MPI tracers will behave under varying excitation field conditions.

We synthesized iron oxide nanoparticles with sizes close to ideal for MPI (ranging from 20-30 nm diameter) and measured their MPI response using a variable frequency magnetic particle spectrometer (MPS) system constructed at the University of Washington. For all measurements, the tracers were coated with an amphiphilic polymer and dispersed in water at a concentration of ~ 1g Fe/L, dilute enough that inter-particle interactions could be neglected. We observed variations in the tracers' magnetic response with both excitation field and frequency; however, the relative magnitude of variation was small. We considered the point spread function (dm/dH, with units m^3) measured by the MPS and also recovered M(H) data by integrating the dm/dH data. Examples are provided for 22 and 25 nm tracers in the figure. We observed hysteresis in the M(H) loops, with a small coercive field that increased with average tracer particle size. For 25 nm tracers, the coercivity was ~3.5 mT/μ_0 when the excitation field amplitude was 20 mT/μ_0 and the frequency 26 kHz. The coercivity increased with amplitude and frequency. For small field amplitudes (~ 5 mT/μ_0), the tracer magnetization was not saturated by each cycle of the excitation field, resulting in a "minor loop." When the field amplitude was increased beyond the amplitude required to saturate the tracer magnetization, the m(H) loop remained relatively unchanged. Varying frequency in the range of 15 to 40 kHz had a smaller effect than varying amplitude (5 to ~50 mT/μ_0), resulting in small changes in coercivity of a few mT/μ_0.

In general, the changes we observed in the tracer response were small for the range of test conditions. Even when only a minor loop was excited, the maximum value of dm/dH was consistent after correcting for the magnetic ramp rate, $B_{max}\omega$. While the field of view of a single excitation is reduced, multiple fields of view could be stitched together to recover the information provided by a larger excitation. We conclude that though excitation field parameters do affect tracer magnetization, optimized MPI tracers will perform well under a variety of applied field conditions and adjustments necessary for patient safety can be made without significant impact on MPI tracer performance.

Corresponding Author: R. M. Ferguson, matt@lodespin.com

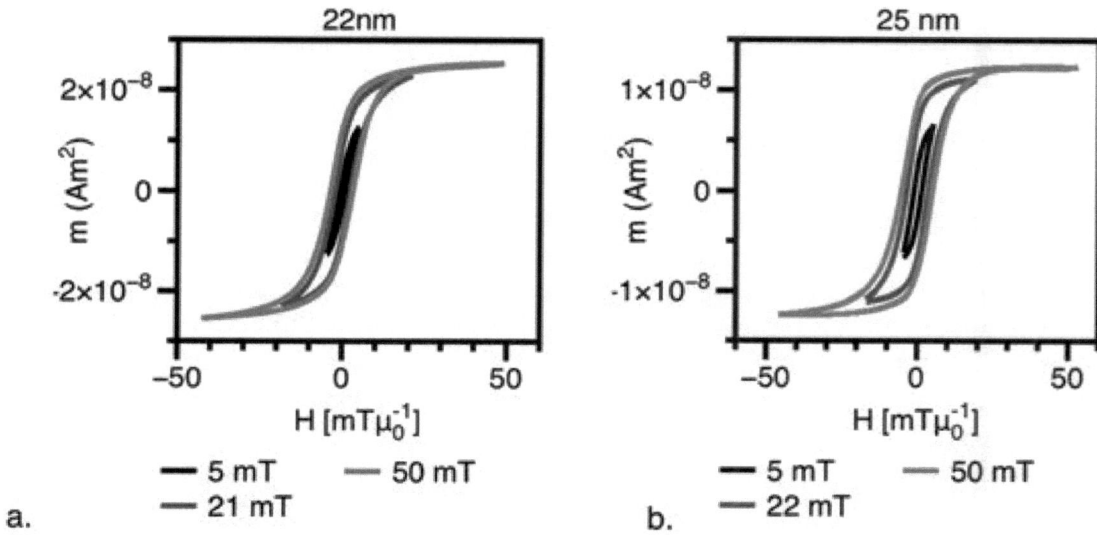

Figure 1. M(H) loops determined by integrating dm/dH data measured with a magnetic particle spectrometer system at the University of Washington. The measurement frequency was fixed at 26 kHz.

Acknowledgements:

This work was supported by the National Institutes of Health's (NIH) grant no. 2R42EB013520-02A1 and NSF grant IIP-1215556

Corresponding Author: R. M. Ferguson, matt@lodespin.com

HYDRODYNAMIC FRACTIONATION TO ENHANCE MPI PERFORMANCE OF RESOVIST®

Norbert Löwa[1], Patrick Knappe[2], Dietmar Eberbeck[1], Andreas F. Thuenemann[2], Lutz Trahms[1]

[1]*Physikalisch-Technische Bundesanstalt, Berlin, Germany*
[2]*Bundesanstalt fuer Materialforschung und -pruefung, Berlin, Germany*

It is well known that the magnetic properties of the tracer material determine the spatial resolution of MPI. Since the invention of MPI, Resovist® has been the most frequently used imaging tracer due to its favorable MPI performance. The reason for that is not yet fully understood due to the very complex formulation of Resovist®. Studies revealed that Resovist® exhibits a bimodal size distribution, consisting of small primary particles, some of which form stable aggregates of twice the radius [1,2]. Attempts to separate the most suitable magnetic particles (MNP) by magnetic separation led to an improvement of MPI signal amplitude by a factor of 2 [3].

In this work we focused on the hydrodynamic separation of Resovist® using asymmetric flow field-flow fractionation (A4F). A4F is based on an elution method where hydrodynamic extension of MNP influences their retention time. The obtained fractions typically reveal a narrow size distribution and permit accurate size evaluation. Here, fractions were collected at intervals of 1 minute for 35 minutes in 6 repetitions. The fractions 14 to 32 were examined further in this study. For subsequent investigation one liquid and one freeze dried sample was prepared from each fraction.

To discriminate between core and hydrodynamic properties of the fractions we investigated the immobilized and liquid samples by magnetorelaxometry (MRX). When deriving size distributions from MRX, we assumed spherical particles with diameters d obeying a log-normal function $f(d)$. We estimated the diameter of the mean volume d_V and the dispersion parameter σ. Information on the anisotropy energy $E_A = K \cdot V$ can be retrieved by analyzing the relaxation of immobilized samples. Here, K is the anisotropy constant and V is the effective magnetic volume of the particles. We found that the anisotropy energy E_A, also determining Néel relaxation, strongly increases from fraction 18 to fraction 25 by 110 %. For fractions of earlier elution times no MRX signal could be measured, due to the fact that smaller particles typically exhibit low anisotropy values and shorter relaxation times which cannot be resolved with our system. These findings strongly correlate with magnetic particle spectroscopy (MPS) results (25 mT magnetic field amplitude, 25 kHz frequency). With regard to those fractions containing small particles (fraction 14 to 17), the difference between the third harmonic amplitudes of fluid and immobilized samples was about 6 %. This means that the magnetic moments follow the external field primarily by Néel processes due to their small anisotropy energy E_A. For fractions of later elution times this gap increased up to 60 %. These results correspond to the phase lag φ measured with MPS, which decreases from $\varphi = -5°$ down to $\varphi = -20°$ with increasing elution time. Regarding the overall MPS signal improvement compared to the original sample, the third harmonic amplitude of fraction 23 increased by factor 2.3.

Using a sample of Resovist®, we demonstrated the potential of improving MPI performance of a MNP preparation by A4F. Furthermore, the characterization of hydrodynamically separated fractions shows that Resovist® exhibits a broad spectrum of anisotropy energies E_A which have a significant influence on the MPS signal. These results are a major step forward towards understanding MPI performance of Resovist®. This is important to design novel MPI tracer materials and could help for further developments of separation techniques.

Corresponding Author: N. Löwa, norbert.loewa@ptb.de

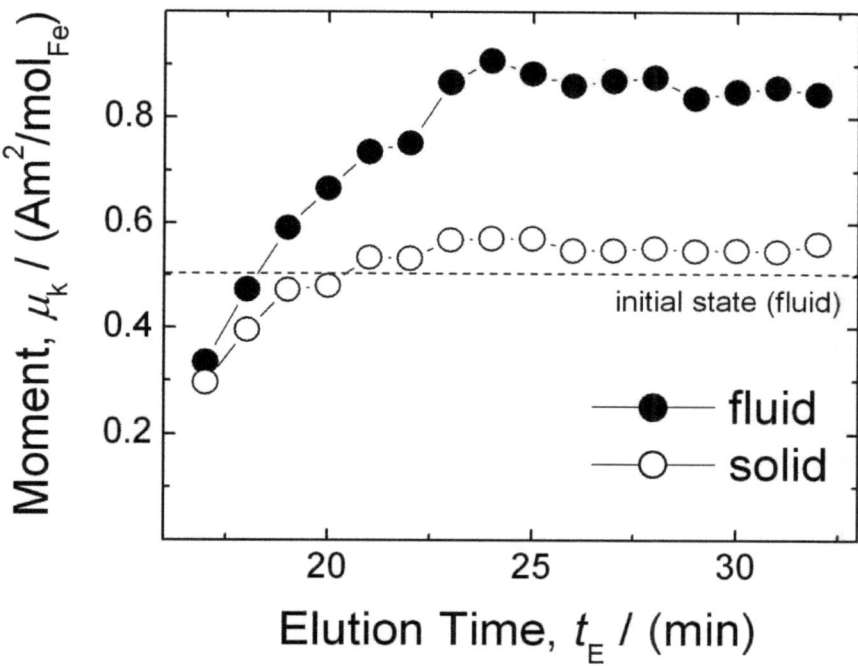

Figure | MPS measurement (B_{excit} = 25 mT, f = 25 kHz) of separated fractions: Amplitude of third harmonic μ_3 normalized to iron content is shown for fraction 17 to 32 in fluid (filled symbols) and solid state (open symbols). It can clearly be seen that the signal increases with elution time up to factor 2.3 compared to the original sample in liquid state.

[1] Thuenemann, Andreas F., et al. "In situ analysis of a bimodal size distribution of superparamagnetic nanoparticles." *Analytical Chemistry* 81.1 (2009): 296-301.

[2] Eberbeck, D., et al. "How the size distribution of magnetic nanoparticles determines their magnetic particle imaging performance." *Applied Physics Letters* 98.18 (2011): 182502-182502.

[3] Löwa, N., et al. "Potential of improving MPI performance by magnetic separation." *Magnetic Particle Imaging*. Springer Berlin Heidelberg, 2012. 73-78.

Corresponding Author: N. Löwa, norbert.loewa@ptb.de

MAGNETIC CHARACTERISATION OF CLUSTERED CORE MAGNETIC NANOPARTICLES FOR MPI

Nicole Gehrke[1], David Heinke[1], Dietmar Eberbeck[2], Frank Ludwig[3], Thilo Wawrzik[3], Christian Kuhlmann[3], Andreas Briel[1]

[1]*nanoPET Pharma GmbH, Berlin, Germany*
[2]*Bioelectricity and Biomagnetism, Physikalisch-Technische Bundesanstalt, Berlin, Germany*
[3]*Institute of Electrical Measurement and Fundamental Electrical Engineering, Technische Universität Braunschweig, Germany*

In previous work[1], we reported on different in-house synthesized iron oxide nanoparticles with seemingly identical structure (overall size, core structure, coating) which, however, surprisingly showed significant differences in their MPI efficacy. The particles with the highest observed efficacy, NPIO-1, exhibited a magnetic particle spectral (MPS) amplitude of up to 10 times higher than NPIO-2, the particles with the lowest efficacy involved in this study, and a 3-fold increased MPS amplitude as compared to the gold-standards Resovist® and FeraSpin™ R[2]. Since the cores of all investigated particles including NPIO-1 and NPIO-2 were comprised of clusters of small-sized crystallites of about 5 nm (so-called multicore particles), we attributed these findings to different interactions between these crystallites within the particles' cores[3]. To explore and identify the potential to further improve the MPI efficacy of such particles, it is desirable to understand the relation between particle structure and particle magnetic properties in more detail. Thus, in the present study, we performed an extensive characterization and analysis of the static and dynamic magnetic properties of these nanoparticles.

We synthesized several batches of the particles NPIO-1 and NPIO-2 by the aqueous precipitation method and performed basic physicochemical characterization on each batch to confirm reproducibility prior to further analysis. For magnetic characterization, liquid as well as freeze-dried, i.e. immobilized, particle samples were prepared. Measurements of the MPS, the complex (ac) susceptibility, the magnetorelaxation (MRX) signal and static magnetization (M(H)-curves) were conducted.

The obtained data and the parameters calculated thereof are presented and discussed. The synthesis and the MPS of the particles were shown to be reproducible. We found that the static and dynamic magnetic properties of the particles are (semi-) quantitatively reflected by their MPS efficacy. Furthermore, the data indicates an interaction between the crystallites within the cores. The degree of this interaction, however, differs significantly between particles NPIO-1 and NPIO-2, despite their similarities between their crystallite size, cluster size as well as overall hydrodynamic size.

Corresponding Author: N. Gehrke, nicole.gehrke@nanopet.de

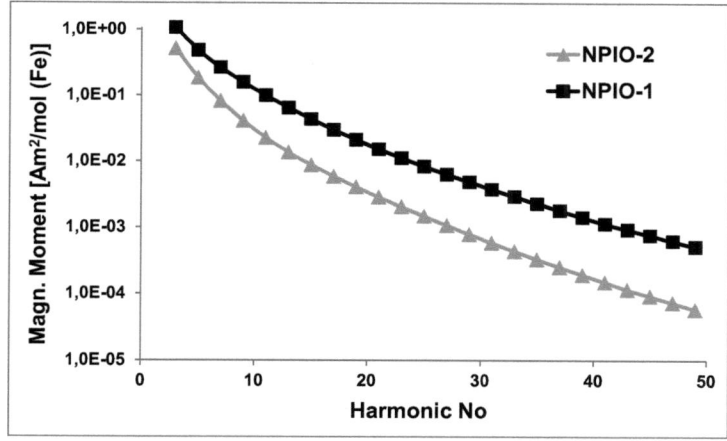

Fig.1: *Main basic particle properties (bottom) and MPS (drive field 25 mT/μ_0, f_0=25.25 kHz) (top) of the particles NPIO-1 and NPIO-2.*

[1] Gehrke et al *"The Potential of Clustered Core Magnetic Particles for MPI"*, IEEE XPlore (2013), DOI 10.1109/IWMPI.2013.6528368)

[2] N. Gehrke et al , "New Perspectives for MPI: A Toolbox for Tracer Research," in: Magnetic Particle Imaging, T. M. Buzug and J. Borgert, Eds., Springer Proceedings in Physics, vol. 140, Springer Berlin Heidelberg (pp. 99-103), March 2012

[3] Lartigue et al "Cooperative Organization in Iron Oxide Multi-Core Nanoparticles Potentiates Their Efficiency as Heating Mediators and MRI Contrast Agents" ACS Nano (2012), 6 (12)

Acknowledgements: This work was supported by the German Federal Ministry of Economics and Technology grant No`s. KF2725002UW2 and KF3061201UW2.

Corresponding Author: N. Gehrke, nicole.gehrke@nanopet.de

TUNING MAGNETIC DIPOLAR INTERACTION FOR ENHANCING MAGNETIC PARTICLE IMAGING PERFORMANCE

Subhasis Sarangi

St. John's Research Institute, St. John's National Academy of Health Sciences, Bangalore, India

The performance of magnetic nanoparticle systems is intimately associated with their composition, size, shape, and magnetic anisotropy. It has been observed that cooperative magnetic behavior of multi-core magnetic nanoparticle systems enhance magnetic particle imaging (MPI) performance over single-core magnetic nanoparticle systems. We propose a theoretical model based on the dipolar interactions between magnetic nanoparticles to understand the underlying mechanism. The model is validated experimentally for both commercially available and laboratory synthesized magnetic nanoparticles using a magnetic particle spectrometer. The model is used to establish a quantitative link between the particle assembling, the interactions and the MPI performance.

Corresponding Author: S. Sarangi, ssarangi@sjri.res.in

TUNING SURFACE COATINGS OF OPTIMIZED MAGNETITE NANOPARTICLE TRACERS FOR IN VIVO MPI

Amit P. Khandhar[1], R. Matthew Ferguson[2], Hamed Arami[1], Scott J. Kemp[2], Kannan M. Krishnan[1]

[1]*Materials Science & Engineering, University of Washington, USA*
[2]*Lodespin Labs, Washington, USA*

Surface coatings provide biocompatibility to superparamagnetic iron oxide nanoparticle (SPIONs) tracers designed for MPI; furthermore, surface coatings play a critical role in preserving the key properties that are responsible for optimum performance in physiological environments. Particularly, surface coatings must (1) preserve the magnetization reversal process of optimized SPIONs in physiological environments and (2) prevent their rapid clearance from blood to enable both first-pass cardiovascular and blood pool imaging. Blood consists a variety of plasma proteins that are responsible for the sequestration of most intravenously (IV) administered materials – when adsorbed to the surface of SPIONs, plasma proteins can induce particle aggregation that is detrimental to both magnetization reversal processes and blood circulation time; thus, surface coatings with non-fouling properties to adequately resist protein adsorption must be developed for MPI tracers.

Here we show the effect of tuning poly(ethylene glycol) (PEG)-based surface coatings on the *in vitro* and *in vivo* (mouse model) MPI performance of SPIONs. Our results showed that varying PEG molecular weight had a profound impact on colloidal stability – characterized using Dynamic Light Scattering (DLS) – and the *m'(H)* response of SPIONs – characterized in a 25 kHz/40 mT$\mu_0^{-1}{}_{p-p}$ Magnetic Particle Spectrometer (MPS); critically, increasing PEG molecular weight from 5 kDa to 20 kDa preserved colloidal stability and *m'(H)* response of 25 nm SPIONs – the optimum core diameter for MPI – in serum-rich cell culture medium for up to 24 hours. Due to the longer chain length of 20K-PEG, the hydrodynamic diameter measured using DLS was 60 nm, which was ~50% greater than SPIONs coated with 5K-PEG. We hypothesized that the longer chain length of 20K-PEG, and the resulting larger hydrodynamic size, provides greater resistance to protein adsorption. Furthermore, *in vivo* circulation studies in mice show that the improved colloidal stability and sustained *m'(H)* response in serum-rich medium translates to a longer blood half-life. Initial studies showed that 20 nm core diameter SPIONs with a 40 nm hydrodynamic diameter have a blood half-life of ~18 minutes, and blood half-life studies with 25 nm core diameter SPIONs coated with the newly developed 20K-PEG are currently underway. We anticipate that the development of MPI SPION tracers with long blood half-lives have potential not only in vascular imaging applications, but also enable opportunities in cancer targeting and imaging – a critical step towards early cancer detection using the new MPI modality.

Acknowledgements: This work was supported by the National Institutes of Health's (NIH) grant no. 2R42EB013520-02A1.

Corresponding Author: A. P. Khandhar, amitk@uw.edu

Session 7

Medical Applications

Chairs: M. Magnani, J. Barkhausen

Keynote

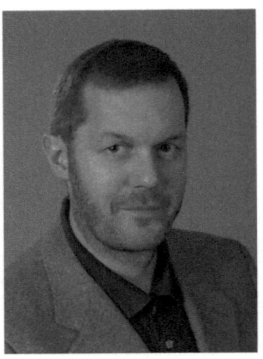

Prof. Matthias Taupitz

Department of Radiology, Charité Berlin, Germany

Challenges for MPI: What are the Requirements a New Diagnostic Tool Must Meet?

STEM CELL VITALITY ASSESSMENT USING MAGNETIC PARTICLE SPECTROSCOPY

Florian Fidler[1], Maria Steinke[2], Alexander Kraupner[3], Cordula Gruettner[4], Karl-Heinz Hiller[1], Andreas Briel[3], Fritz Westphal[4], Heike Walles[2], Peter Michael Jakob[1]

[1]*Research Center Magnetic-Resonance-Bavaria, Würzburg, Germany*
[2]*Fraunhofer Institute for Interfacial Engineering and Biotechnolgy IGB, Tissue Engineering and Regenerative Medicine, Würzburg, Germany*
[3]*nanoPet Pharma GmbH, Berlin, Germany*
[4]*Micromod GmbH, Rostock-Warnemuende, Germany*

Human mesenchymal stem cells (hMSCs) are a promising tool in regenerative medicine. Cell homing of cells labeled with iron oxide nanoparticles can be tracked with various modalities like magnetic particle imaging (MPI) or magnetic resonance imaging (MRI). Beside cell homing at the targeted organ, assessing the cell vitality is of paramount during the healing process. In this study we present our first results in monitoring the cell vitality based on magnetic particle spectroscopy (MPS) findings.

In total three different magnetic nanoparticles, N1C with carboxydextran coating, M3A and M4A with dextran coating were used for stem cell labeling. On top M3A and M4A particles were additionally coated with poly-L-lysine (PLL) in order to facilitate iron uptake. The applied labeling protocol leads to a significant increase in cell's iron content without affecting the cell viability. In all MPS experiments 250k cells were measured in 50µl solution using a home build magnetic particle spectrometer which is able to operate at 10 kHz to 25 kHz with field strength up to 40 mT. The probe temperature was stabilized to 37°C during measurement; additionally a home build temperature stabilized vortex unit for probe preparation was used. The spectrometer was calibrated for quantitative measurements and was able to detect magnetic moments down to $2*10^{-10}$ Am^2.

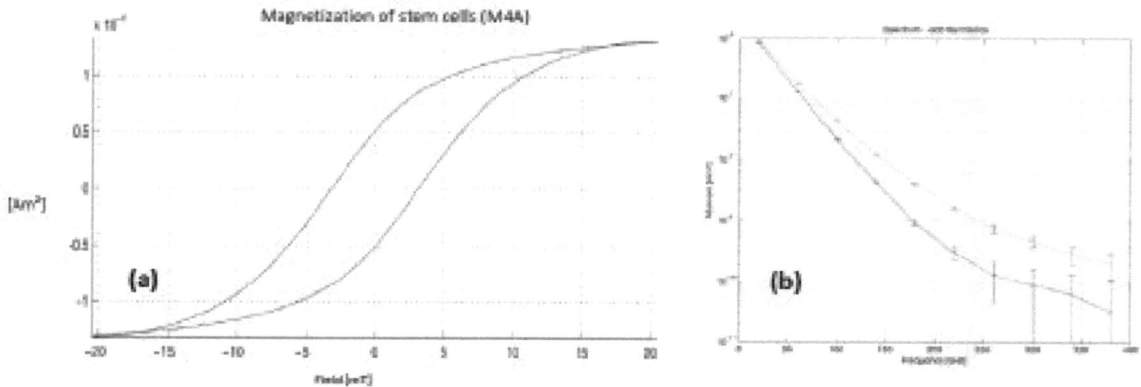

Fig.1: (a) Measured magnetization curve of intact labeled stem cells. The shown cells are labeled with M4A particles at 37°C. (b) Example spectrum (only odd Harmonics shown) of intact (black line) and degraded (gray line) stem cells labeled with N1C particles measured at 20 kHz and 37°C. The degradation process was continuously monitored (not shown here).

For cell vitality assessment MPS spectra were continuously monitored during a cell degradation process initiated by adding sodium dodecyl sulfate (SDS) to the probes, which dissolves the cells.
During this dissolution experiment the MPS spectra showed a specific change in the higher-order harmonics, which can be attributed to a change in Brownian relaxation.

Corresponding Author: F. Fidler, fidler@mr-bavaria.de

These findings suggest, that well designed iron-oxide nanoparticles not only can be used as a reporter for cell homing, but also for cell viability.

In summary, these findings also indicate the potential to estimate the cell vitality in the *in vivo* scenario.

Acknowledgements: This work was supported by the EU FP7 HEALTH program (IDEA – "Identification, homing and monitoring of therapeutic cells for regenerative medicine – Identify, Enrich, Accelerate")

Corresponding Author: F. Fidler, fidler@mr-bavaria.de

MAGNETIC PARTICLE IMAGING (MPI): VISUALIZATION AND QUANTIFICATION OF VASCULAR STENOSIS PHANTOMS

Julian Haegele[1], Jürgen Rahmer[2], Robert Duschka[1], Catharina Schaecke[1], Nicolaos Panagiotopoulos[1], Julia Tonak[1], Jörn Borgert[2], Joerg Barkhausen[1], Florian M. Vogt[1]

[1]*Clinic for Radiology and Nuclear Medicine, University Hospital Schleswig Holstein Lübeck, Germany*
[2]*Forschungslaboratorien, Philips Technologie, Innovative Technologies, Hamburg, Germany*

Magnetic Particle Imaging (MPI) is seen as a promising method for cardiovascular imaging and guidance of cardiovascular interventions [1, 2]. This rests upon its good spatial resolution, very high temporal resolution, sensitivity and signal to noise ratio. As the strength of the MPI-signal is proportional to the amount of superparamagnetic iron oxide nanoparticles (SPIOs), MPI is an inherent quantitative imaging method [1]. This can be a valuable tool in evaluating the extent of pathologies like vascular stenosis and in therapy control. Purpose of this study was to visualize and quantify different vascular stenosis phantoms using MPI.

Nine standardized stenosis-phantoms were used, each featuring a circular lumen of 10 mm diameter. The lumen of the phantoms narrowed conically to a residual lumen of 1 mm diameter amounting to a 99 % stenosis of the cross section of the normal diameter, 2 mm (96 %), 3 mm (91 %), 4 mm (84 %), 5 mm (75 %), 6 mm (64 %), 7 mm (51 %), 8 mm (36 %) or 9mm (19 %), respectively. For MPI, the phantoms were filled with a 1% and 5% dilution of Resovist (Bayer Pharma AG), corresponding to 0.28 and 1.4 mg(Fe)/ml Resovist, respectively. Images were acquired using a pre-clinical MPI-demonstrator (Philips Research, Hamburg, Germany, field of view 36 x 36 x 20 mm^3, temporal resolution 46 Volumes per second, corresponding to [3]). Imaging was conducted in steady state without flow and during manual movement of the phantoms through the field of view of the MPI-demonstrator. Beside image reconstruction, the MPI-signal was used for intensity measurements to quantify the grade of stenosis. For comparison, the same stenosis-phantoms were evaluated with contrast-enhanced CT (Siemens Definition AS64, 12 % Imeron 300 (Bracco Imaging)) and MRI (Philips Achieva 1.5 T, 3 % Gadovist (Bayer Vital). Acquisition time for the 3D CT, MRI, and MPI scans was 1.2 s, 60 s, and 21 ms, respectively.

With a resulting spatial resolution of about 3 x 3 x 1 mm^3, MPI was able to visualize all residual lumina of the stenoses accurately except for the highest grade stenosis (1 mm, 99 %). Additionally, MPI was able to detect the residual lumen of the 1 mm (99 %) stenosis using the MPI-signal. It was possible to quantify the extent of the stenoses down to 6 mm (64 %) independently of the Resovist concentration and the rate of movement of the stenosis-phantoms through the field of view. Higher grade stenoses were underestimated, the stenosis of 84% was measured as 74 %, 91 % as 79 %, 96 % as 82 % and 99 % as 88 %. CT exhibited the highest spatial resolution, followed by MRI; both modalities were able to visualize all stenoses. Direct quantification of vascular stenoses using MPI is possible in phantoms with very low concentrations of Resovist. Due to the high temporal resolution of the system, visualization and quantification is independent of the movement of the probe, which may be beneficial for future clinical applications where respiratory and cardiac motion occur. With current experimental MPI-systems and available tracer materials, the spatial resolution at high imaging speeds is limited, so that high grade stenoses are underestimated systematically due to a partial volume effect. However, in this phantom study, the MPI-signal of small structures like residual lumina in high grade vascular stenoses is still detectable, even if the spatial resolution is too low for visualization or reliable signal quantification. This may allow differentiation of high grade stenoses and vascular obliteration.

Corresponding Author: J. Haegele, julian.haegele@uksh.de

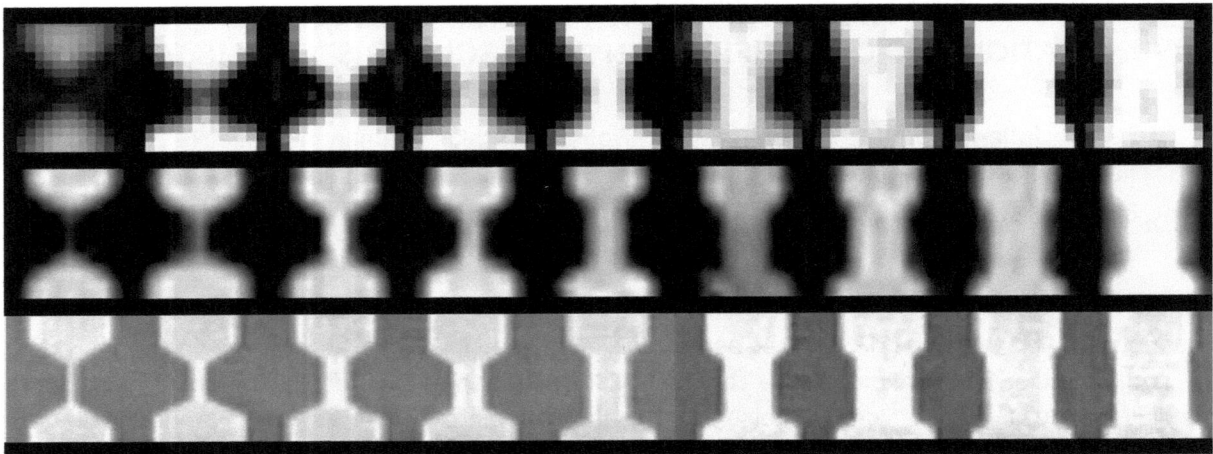

Fig. 1: MPI (top), MRI (middle) and CT (bottom) in comparison. CT exhibits the highest spatial resolution. In MPI, the lumen of the highest grade stenosis (1 mm) is hardly delineable.

[1] Borgert J, Schmidt JD, Schmale I, et al. Fundamentals and applications of magnetic particle imaging. J Cardiovasc Comput Tomogr. 2012;6:149-53. doi:10.1016/j.jcct.2012.04.007.

[2] Goodwill PW, Saritas EU, Croft LR, et al. X-Space MPI: Magnetic Nanoparticles for Safe Medical Imaging. Adv Mater. 2012;24:3870-7. doi:DOI 10.1002/adma.201200221.

[3] Haegele J, Rahmer J, Gleich B, et al. Magnetic Particle Imaging: Visualization of Instruments for Cardiovascular Intervention. Radiology. 2012;265:933-8. doi:DOI 10.1148/radiol.12120424.

Corresponding Author: J. Haegele, julian.haegele@uksh.de

TIME-EVOLUTION CONTRAST OF TARGET MRI USING ANTIBODY FUNCTIONALIZED MAGNETIC NANOPARTICLES: AN ANIMAL MODEL

S.Y. Yang[1], H.E. Horng[2], J.J. Chieh[2], C.C. Wu[3,4], K.W. Huang[5,6], H.C. Yang[7]

[1]MagQu Co., Ltd. Taiwan
[2]Institute of Electro-Optical Science and Technology, National Taiwan Normal University, Taiwan
[3]Department of Internal Medicine, National Taiwan University Hospital, College of Medicine, National Taiwan University, Taiwan
[4]Department of Primary Care Medicine, National Taiwan National Taiwan University, Taiwan
[5]Department of Surgery & Hepatitis Research Center, National Taiwan University Hospital, Taiwan
[6]Graduate Institute of Clinical Medicine, College of Medicine, National Taiwan University, Taiwan
[7]Department of Electro-optical Engineering, Kun Shan University, Taiwan

Due to the non-toxicity and versatilities in surface bio-functions, Fe_3O_4 magnetic nanoparticles are applied to *in-vivo* target labeling and are mapped using medical imaging instruments. In this work, high-quality antibody functionalized Fe_3O_4 magnetic nanoparticles are synthesized [1]. Such characterizations as particle morphology, particle size, stability, magnetization, relaxivity of magnetic particles are investigated [2,3]. The results show that the mean diameter of antibody functionalized magnetic nanoparticles is around 55 nm, and the relaxivity of the magnetic particles is 145 $(mM·s)^{-1}$. In addition to characterizing the magnetic nanoparticles, the feasibility of using the antibody functionalized magnetic nanoparticles for the contrast medium of target magnetic resonance imaging is investigated. These antibody functionalized magnetic nanoparticles are injected into rats bearing with tumor. The tumor magnetic-resonance image becomes darker after the injection, and then recovers 40 hours after the injection [4], as shown in Fig. 1. The tumor magnetic-resonance image becomes darkest at around 20 hours after the injection. As a comparison, the time-evolution magnetic resonance images are taken in case of the injection of magnetic nanoparticles without antibody into rats. It was found that the darken effect of the tumor magnetic-resonance image occurs after the injection, however disappears 20 hours after the injection. Thus, the observing time window for the specific labeling of tumors with antibody functionalized magnetic nanoparticles was found to be 20 hours after injecting bio-functionalized magnetic nanoparticles into rats. The biopsy of tumor is stained after the injection to evidence that the long-term darkness of tumor magnetic-resonance image is due to the specific anchoring of antibody functionalized magnetic nanoparticles at tumor. Meanwhile, the metabolism of injected Fe_3O_4 magnetic nanoparticles in rats is studied [5].

[1] S.Y. Yang, Z.F. Jian, H.E. Horng, Chin-Yih Hong, H.C. Yang, C.C Wu, and Y.H. Lee, "Dual immobilization and magnetic manipulation of magnetic nanoparticles", J. Magn. Magn. Mater. 320, 2688 (2008).

[2] C.Y. Hong, W.H. Chen, Z.F. Jian, S.Y. Yang, H.E. Horng, L.C. Yang, and H.C. Yang, "Wash-free immunomagnetic detection for serum through magnetic susceptibility reduction", Appl. Phys. Lett. 90, 74105 (2007).

[3] C.C. Wu, L.Y. Lin, L.C. Lin, H.C. Huang, Y.B. Liu, M.C. Tsai, Y.L. Gao, W.C. Wang, S.Y. Yang, H.E. Horng, H.C. Yang, W.K. Tseng, T.L. Lee, C.F. Hsuan, and Isaac W.Y. Tseng, "Bio-functionalized magnetic nanoparticles for in-vitro labeling and in-vivo locating specific bio-molecules", Appl. Phys. Lett. 92, 142504 (2008).

[4] K.W. Huang, J.J. Chieh, H.E. Horng, C.Y. Hong, and H.C. Yang, "Characteristics of magnetic labeling on liver tumors with anti-alpha-fetoprotein-mediated Fe_3O_4 magnetic nanoparticles", Intl. J. Nanomed. 7, 2987 (2012).

Corresponding Author: S.Y. Yang, syyang@magqu.com

[5] W.K. Tseng, J.J. Chieh, Y.F. Yang, C.K. Chiang, Y.L. Chen, S.Y. Yang, H.E. Horng, H.C. Yang, and C.C. Wu, "A noninvasive method to determine the fate of Fe3O4 nanoparticles following intravenous injection using scanning SQUID biosusceptometry", PLOS one 7, e48510 (2012).

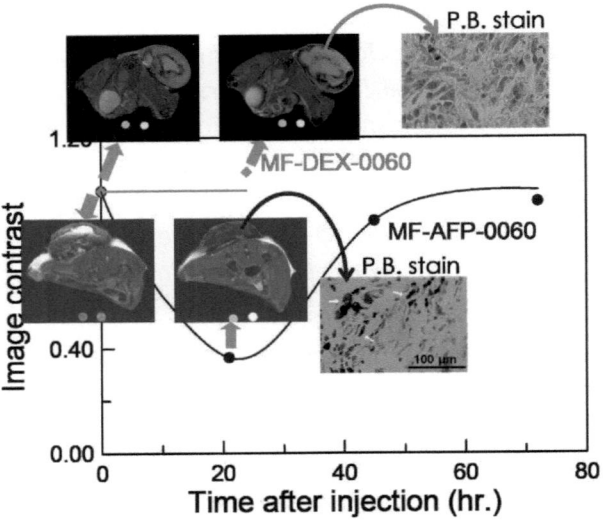

Fig. 1. Time-evolution contrast MRI using magnetic nanoparticles.

Corresponding Author: S.Y. Yang, syyang@magqu.com

IN VIVO MPI NEURAL CELL MONITORING IN THE RAT BRAIN

Bo Zheng[1], Tandis Vazin[2], Patrick Goodwill[1], David Schaffer[1,2], Steven Conolly[1,3]

[1]Department of Bioengineering, University of California, Berkeley, USA
[2]Department of Chemical and Biomolecular Engineering, University of California, Berkeley, USA
[3]Department of Electrical Engineering and Computer Science, Berkeley, USA

Introduction: The development of cell-based therapies has been hampered by the lack of pre-clinical imaging techniques suitable for tracking therapeutic cell implants. Magnetic Particle Imaging (MPI) has shown great promise for long-term tracking of magnetically labeled cells in vivo [1-2]. Unlike existing techniques, MPI images of cells labeled with superparamagnetic iron oxide (SPIOs) are not obscured by surrounding anatomy. Previously, we demonstrated that MPI creates positive-contrast images of labeled human embryonic stem cell (hESC)-derived cells sensitivity of 500-1000 cells/voxel [unpublished]. In this work, we describe the proof-of-concept MPI monitoring of labeled neural cell implants in the rat brain over a therapeutically relevant time scale.

Methods: After stereotactically implanting 0.5 million labeled hESC-derived neural progenitor cells in three immunosuppressed Fischer 344 rats, we tracked the grafts using a projection-format MPI imager over a 12-week period. Postmortem MRI images at 7T were taken of the animal brains, with histological confirmation of iron via Prussian blue staining and immunostaining.

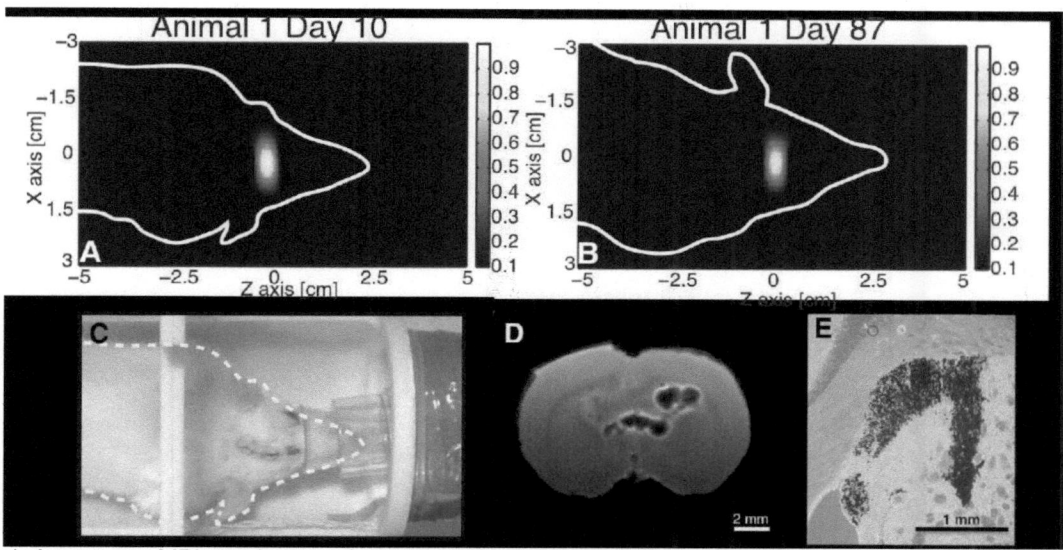

Figure 1. Long-term MPI monitoring of neural implants. (A) and (B) show MPI images of SPIO-labeled neural progenitor cell grafts from the same animal at 10 and 87 days after implantation, with photo reference (C). The total MPI signal from the cell graft showed no significant clearance of SPIOs within 12 weeks. (FOV: 6 cm x 10 cm, 10 second scan time). (D) shows a proton-weighted zero-echo time (ZTE) MRI postmortem coronal image. SPIO-labeled cells are visible along the cortex but are hard to distinguish from other anatomical features. Image acquired on a Bruker 7T scanner with 2.56 cm³ FOV, 0.1 um³ voxel size, and 20 min scan time. (E) shows Prussian-blue stained SPIOs present in the cell graft in the needle track and toward the ventricle.

Results: The grafts were readily discernible in MPI images, producing excellent positive contrast in the brain with no interference from other signal sources (Fig. 1A-B). For comparison, we show postmortem coronal slices of the same SPIO-labeled cell graft in a 7T MRI (Fig. 1C). A postmortem MRI image (Fig. 1D) shows excellent localization of the cell graft at the injection side. When we quantified the total MPI signal from the cell grafts over time, we saw no significant clearance of the SPIO label over 12 weeks (Fig. 1B), which was confirmed by histology (Fig. 1E) using Prussian blie staining, MRI, and

Corresponding Author: B. Zheng, bozheng@berkeley.edu

immunohistochemistry. A control animal injected with an equivalent amount of Resovist showed no MPI signal from 4 days post-injection.

Discussion: Here we demonstrate the first long-term cell implant monitoring using MPI. We note that while the negative contrast in MRI makes it difficult to accurately quantify cell number or differentiate between SPIOs and other anatomy or image artifacts, MPI is able to unambiguously determine the location and number of the cell implant. Hence, the high specificity and quantification in MPI greatly complements the excellent resolution and anatomical reference in MRI for highly accurate and informational noninvasive cell tracking. Indeed, there already the exist efforts to combine the two modalities into a dedicated system [4]. These techniques may efficiently accelerate the development of many cell therapies on the clinical horizon.

[1] J. W. M. Bulte et al., Proc IWMPI 2010, pp. 201-204.

[2] A. Antonelli et al., Magnetic Particle Imaging, vol. 140, no. Springer Proceedings in Physics, pp. 175-179, 2012.

[3] B. Zheng et al., Proc. IWMPI 2013, vol. 104, no. 435, pp. 1-1.

[4] J. Franke et al., Proc. IWMPI 2013, DOI: 10.1109/IWMPI.2013.6528363.

Corresponding Author: B. Zheng, bozheng@berkeley.edu

Session 8

Magnetic Particle Imaging II

Chairs: U. Heinen, D. Baumgarten

FLOW ASSESSMENT FROM IN VITRO AND IN SILICO DYNAMIC MPI DATA

Romain Lacroix[1], Jürgen Rahmer[2], Oliver M. Weber[2], Hernan G. Morales[1], Sherif Makram-Ebeid[1]

[1]Philips Research Paris, France
[2]Philips Research Hamburg, Germany

MPI has shown great potential in imaging small anatomical structures such as vessels and organs in mice [1][2]. Its high acquisition speed and fine data resolution make MPI a serious candidate for quantification tasks, including real time blood flow imaging. For the moment, the MPI system is not fully developed and few in-vivo data are available. To circumvent this problem, we propose in-vitro and in-silico flow experiments.

We injected a bolus of nanoparticles inside an in-vitro phantom, extracted the flow of tracer and estimated the average flow rate using an optical flow method. This experiment was performed in the preclinical MPI demonstrator available at Philips Research facilities in Hamburg. Single volume acquisitions were performed inside this phantom, in which a mixture of water and 1/20 diluted Resovist® was injected. The amount of water-contrast mixture flowing in the phantom inlet was controlled with a straightway diaphragm valve powered with a Lego Mindstorm® unit. During the calibration, the average flow rate was evaluated from a graduated container, and a mean velocity of 32 $cm.s^{-1}$ in the phantom inlet was derived. After acquisition, reconstruction and post-processing, a spatial propagation of the particles was observable inside the phantom.

Afterwards, the phantom lumen was numerically reconstructed and computational fluid dynamics (CFD) simulations were performed to mimic the same propagation process. The CFD software OpenFOAM® was used to reproduce the in-vitro experiment. A surface mesh was generated from manual thresholding on the original MPI data. Flow was assumed to be steady with an average velocity of 32 $cm.s^{-1}$ at the inlet of the CFD model. For the contrast transport in the CFD model, an intensity curve from the in-vitro experiment was extracted and imposed as boundary condition. For the flow estimation in both experiments, state-of-the art techniques of regularized optical flow methods were used. Additionally, the influence of resolution on optical flow accuracy was studied by testing simpler geometries (straight tubes) where the analytical solution is known.

Our optical flow based algorithm yields good qualitative results on the in-vitro phantom (Figure 1). The computed velocity magnitudes in each branch lie in an acceptable range of [5-26] $cm.s^{-1}$, with an average of 14.5 $cm.s^{-1}$ matching well with the known average velocity magnitude (16 $cm.s^{-1}$). However, the accuracy in all areas of the phantom is not guaranteed. Unlike CFD simulations, where resolution can be chosen, MPI has a limited resolution of 1mm. In our in-vitro phantom, 4mm-diameter tubes were used, and optical flow and spatial gradient estimation were roughly approximated and subjected to image blurring, partial volume effect and/or reconstruction artifacts. Further studies on simpler geometries conducted with CFD showed that finer resolutions (0.5 mm, 0.25mm, 0.125mm) can improve the optical flow accuracy (median error <5% for the velocity magnitude).

CFD simulations and in-vitro phantom experiments are necessary to further understand the propagation process of the MPI tracer. The in-vitro experiment proves the possibility to estimate realistic flow patterns with a fast contrast injection. The accuracy can be significantly improved by using CFD models with finer resolutions. Until MPI systems get improved, in-vitro experiment together with in-silico models can provide a valuable help for the assessment of MPI blood flow estimation methods.

Corresponding Author: R. Lacroix, romain.lacroix@philips.com

[1] Three-dimensional real-time in vivo magnetic particle imaging. J Weizenecker et al 2009 Phys. Med. Biol. 54 L1

[2] Nano-particle encapsulation in red blood cells enables bloodpool magnetic particle imaging hours after injection. J Rahmer et al 2013 Phys. Med. Biol. 58 3965

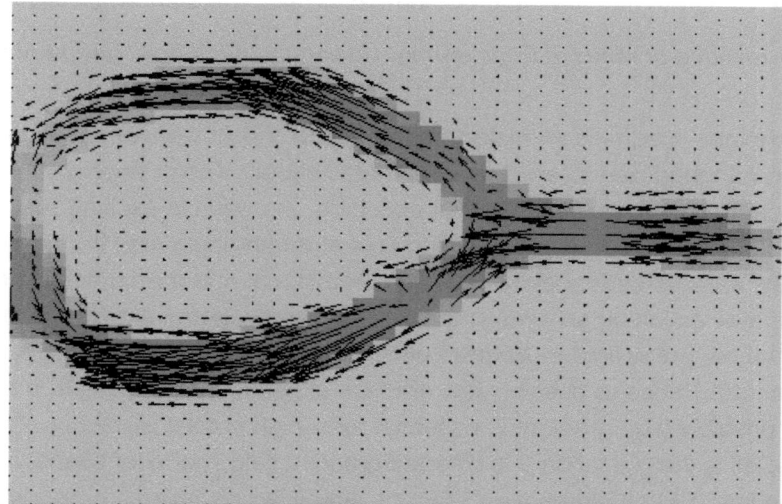

Figure 1 – optical flow estimation in a Y-shape phantom. Arrows represent estimated velocity vectors and grey-scale map is the contrast intensity

TWO DIMENSIONAL MAGNETIC PARTICLE IMAGING WITH A DYNAMIC FIELD FREE LINE SCANNER

Klaas Bente, Matthias Weber, Matthias Gräser, Mandy Ahlborg, Anselm v. Gladiss, Ksenija Gräfe, Gael Bringout, Marlitt Erbe, Timo F. Sattel, Thorsten M. Buzug

Institute of Medical Engineering, University of Lübeck, Germany

In the imaging technique Magnetic Particle Imaging (MPI) the non-linear magnetization behavior of superparamagnetic nanoparticles is used to generate a signal, whose energy is directly proportional to the particle concentration. To achieve spatial encoding, the particle exciting magnetic field typically features a field free point (FFP) and an increasing field strength originating from that point in all spatial directions. This way, a linear dependency of the emitted signal and the particle location is given. The drawback of this spatial encoding scheme is that the measured signal strength is inverse proportional to the gradient of the magnetic field in all three dimensions, while the spatial resolution is proportional to the gradient strength. Hence, a possibly low gradient is necessary to achieve a high signal to noise ratio (SNR), but a possibly high gradient is essential for a high spatial resolution. An important step to cope with this trade-off is the utilization of a different gradient field shape for spatial encoding. If the field features a field free line (FFL) instead of an FFP, the signal is only inverse proportional to the gradient strength in two dimensions, since the gradient in one direction equals zero. This, in fact, means that the area in which particles generate a signal is enlarged without decreasing the gradient strength and the resolution. However, one dimension for spatial encoding is lost, but can be compensated by rotating the FFL over the field of view (FOV), which enables a Radon-based reconstruction [1].

The idea and the principle realization of an electrical rotatable FFL have already been elaborated [2]. The feasibility of image reconstruction with experimentally acquired FFL-MPI data could also be shown [3]. However, due to hardware challenges an FFL-MPI scanner with a rotation of the FFL could not be implemented until today. Such a first scanner is presented here. A short overview over the hardware implementation is presented. The scanner has a bore diameter of 3 cm and a gradient of 1.08 T/m. The optimized scanner design features excellent field quality and enables imaging in a circular field of view limited by the bore diameter.

The main focus lies on the used x-space reconstruction algorithm and the resulting images. All relevant characteristics concerning the acquired raw data, such as sensitivity and SNR, and concerning the reconstructed images, such as resolution, are discussed.

[1] Knopp, T., Erbe, M., Sattel, T. F., Biederer, S., and Buzug, T. M.: A Fourier slice theorem for magnetic particle imaging using a field-free line. *Inverse Problems*, vol. 27, no. 9, , 2011

[2] Knopp, T., Erbe, M., Biederer, S., Sattel, T., and Buzug, T.: Efficient generation of a magnetic field-free line. *Medical Physics*, vol. 37, no. 7, pp. 3538-3540, 2010

[3] Patrick W. Goodwill, Justin J. Konkle, Bo Zheng, Emine U. Saritas, and Steven M. Conolly: Projection X-Space Magnetic Particle Imaging. IEEE Transactions on Medical Imaging, vol. 31, no. 5, pp. 1076-1085, 2012

Corresponding Author: K. Bente, bente@imt.uni-Lübeck.de

CONCEPT OF A GENERATOR FOR THE SELECTION- AND FOCUS FIELD OF A CLINICAL MPI SCANNER

Claas Bontus[1], Bernhard Gleich[1], Bernd David[1], Oliver Mende[2], Jörn Borgert[1]

[1]*Philips Technologie GmbH, Innovative Technologies, Research Laboratories, Hamburg, Germany*
[2]*Philips Medical Systems DMC, Hamburg, Germany*

The selection- and focus field (SeFo field) is an inhomogeneous field with a field free point (FFP) at a specified position. Building a large SeFo field generator for whole-body MPI encompasses a number of challenges. First, the gradient field strength in the vicinity of the FFP must be large enough for obtaining sufficient spatial resolution. Second, the space covered by possible positions of the FFP must be large enough to build up a suitable field of view (FOV). Third, changing positions of the FFP must be possible fast enough to support reasonable temporal resolution. Additionally, the field generator must provide sufficient space to take up the drive-field (DF) generator and still leave enough space for the FOV. Adequate shielding is required for preventing the DF from interacting with the SeFo generator.

We present a concept of a SeFo field generator consisting of 16 channels. Each channel has an electromagnetic coil connected to a current amplifier. Each coil has a core made from soft magnetic material (SMM), i.e. FeSi. Furthermore, SMM is used for field guidance. The central four coils are aligned axially on the vertical (z-)axis. They can be used for generating an FFP and moving it along the z-axis. The remaining twelve channels are arranged on two circles around the inner coils with six coils each. These twelve channels primarily serve for moving the FFP along x and y.

The chosen concept is analyzed by simulations. In particular, we used finite element software (FEM) for addressing the three challenges mentioned above. The input parameters of each simulation are the power consumptions in each coil, resulting in 16 free parameters. Assuming an effective resistance of the copper windings within the coils, the power consumptions are related to current densities. With this approach we can assure that the total power consumption never exceeds a given limit, and we can specify maximum power consumptions for each coil. By variation of the parameters we were able to show that an FFP with gradient field strength of at least 2 T/m should be realizable within a FOV with a diameter of 200 mm. The speed at which the FFP can be moved (slew rate) depends on the inductance of the coils. For obtaining estimates of the various inductances, we used an approach based on the energy stored in the magnetic field. The inductances also depend on the amount of saturation of the SMM. Hence, the slew rate must be determined separately for individual cases.

Corresponding Author: C. Bontus, claas.bontus@philips.com

ULTRA HIGH RESOLUTION MPI

Patrick Vogel[1,2], Martin A. Rückert[1], Peter M. Jakob[1,2], Volker C. Behr[1]

[1]*Department of Experimental Physics 5 (Biophysics), University of Würzburg, Germany*
[2]*Research Center for Magnetic Resonance Bavaria e.V. (MRB), Würzburg, Germany*

Since the first publication of MPI several scanner designs have been presented [1][2][3]. All these scanners operate at gradient strength of about 2-7 T/m, which results in a spatial resolution of about 1 mm [4]. This is a reasonable value for a small animal scanner. For more detailed information about a used particle system which can be of interest for particle design and a better simulation model, it is sometimes necessary to measure at much higher gradient strength and different excitation frequencies. Using two permanent ring-magnets with an inner bore size of 6 mm, which are placed at a distance of 4 mm facing each other with the same pole, a field gradient in the center of about 50 T/m can be generated (fig. 1 (1)). Two additional permanent ring-magnets, which are mounted on a freely moveable rod, stabilize the sample in the middle (fig. 1 (2)). The receive coil is placed inside the main magnets surrounding the sample (fig. 1 (3)). A positioning-coil can move the rod, which holds the sample, relatively to the main magnets (and the receive coil) with different frequencies periodically through the static field gradient of the setup. This approach does not require filter in the receive chain for suppressing the excitation frequency. The only signal, that is induced in the receive coil stems from the sample. This results in a very high sensitivity.

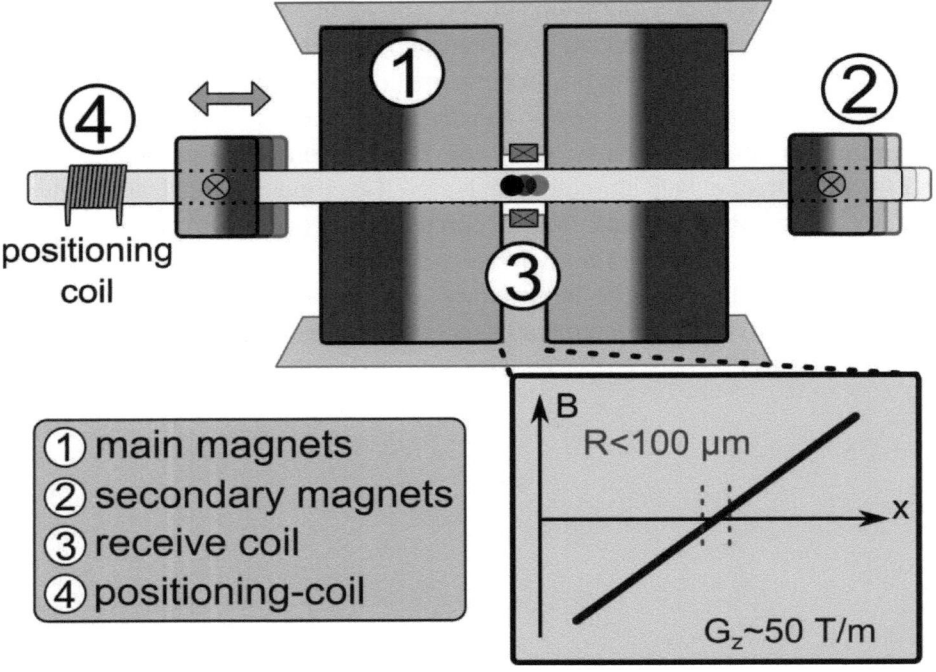

Fig. 1 (1) Two permanent ring-magnets facing each other with the same pole generate a strong field gradient. (2) Secondary permanent ring-magnets stabilize the sample. (3) Receive coil surrounding the sample. (4) A positioning-coil for the sample movement at different frequencies. This setup provides a theoretical resolution of R<100 μm.

Corresponding Author: P. Vogel, Patrick.Vogel@physik.uni-Würzburg.de

With a field gradient of about 50 T/m a theoretical spatial resolution of about 50 µm can be achieved in one direction (calculated with magnetite with 30 nm diameter) [4]. This can be sufficient enough for imaging a single stem cell prepared with Resovist® (Bayer Schering, Germany).

The simple structure of this scanner approach provides a high sensitivity because of the static field and yields the possibility of a simple and cheap high resolution MPS/MPI scanner for ex-vivo samples.

[1] B. Gleich, and J. Weizenecker, "Tomographic imaging using the nonlinear response of magnetic particles", Nature 435, 1214-1217, Jun. 2005.

[2] P. Vogel et al. „Traveling Wave Magnetic Particle Imaging", IEEE TMI, 2013, Doi: 10.1109/TMI.2013.2285472.

[3] P. W. Goodwill et al. "An x-space magnetic particle imaging scanner", Rev. Sci. Instrum., 83, 033708, 2012.

[4] P. W. Goodwill, and S. M. Conolly, "The x-space Formulation of the Magnetic Particle Imaging process", IEEE TMI, vol. 29(11), pp. 1851-1859, 2010.

Corresponding Author: P. Vogel, Patrick.Vogel@physik.uni-Würzburg.de

POSTER

Session I: Friday, March 28

Session II: Saturday, March 29

Poster

Magnetic Particle Imaging

P01 EFFICIENT GRADIENT FIELDS IN MAGNETIC PARTICLE IMAGING – FROM ONE DIMENSION TO MULTIPLE DIMENSIONS

Christian Kaethner[1], Tobias Knopp[2], Mandy Ahlborg[1], Timo F. Sattel[3], Thorsten M. Buzug[1]

[1]Institute of Medical Engineering, Universität zu Lübeck, Germany
[2]Thorlabs GmbH, Lübeck, Germany
[3]Philips Medical Systems DMC GmbH, Hamburg, Germany

Magnetic Particle Imaging (MPI) is a quantitative imaging technique based on magnetic fields [1]. When implementing an MPI system, (resistive) power losses are one of the most limiting factors [2]. These losses limit the achievable gradient strength in the area of the field free point (FFP). This in turn affects the resulting image quality since the gradient strength directly influences the image resolution. Due to the fact that the gradient strength is connected to the spatial resolution of a reconstructed image, a correlation between the spatial resolution and the power loss is given as well. In the following, two different coil configurations to generate a magnetic gradient field are presented. The conventional way is to use a pair of opposing electromagnetic coils carrying currents in opposite directions. This configuration, known as Maxwell coil setup, provides an efficient way to generate the FFP at the center position between both coils. A different way to generate such a gradient field is to arrange two electromagnetic coils, differing in their diameter, concentrically in the same plane. This asymmetric coil arrangement is known as single-sided configuration [3]. With opposing currents, there are two FFPs generated on the common coil axis, one on each side of the coils. However, only the FFP in front of the assembly is used for imaging. Similar to the Maxwell setup, there is an FFP position providing the least power consumption in the single-sided setup, i.e. directly in front of the assembly with a close distance to the coils. Since, the applied coil currents are considered to be constant, the FFP is established only at one certain position. A one-dimensional movement of the FFP can be realized by superimposing alternating currents to at least one coil of the considered setups. However, such a movement requires huge power consumption, if the FFP is shifted considerably off the center position in the Maxwell setup or away from the coils in the single-sided coil assembly, respectively. An approach to generate a magnetic gradient field efficiently with arbitrary axial positioning of the FFP was published recently [4]. The setup proposed in the referred work combines the aforementioned coil arrangements to a hybrid setup consisting of two concentrically arranged coils on opposite sides of the field of view. An optimization of the applied currents combined with the hybrid coil arrangement provides a low-power solution for a one-dimensional FFP movement. However, it is not obviously given that the derived mathematical solution is extendable to two or even three dimensions. In this contribution, it is shown that the efficient gradient field generation can be extended to multiple dimensions. In addition to the derivation of the mathematical formulas, first simulation results will be presented, showing the potential of this approach (see Figure 1). The findings of this extension are an important step to realize human sized MPI scanning devices.

Corresponding Author: C. Kaethner, kaethner@imt.uni-Lübeck.de

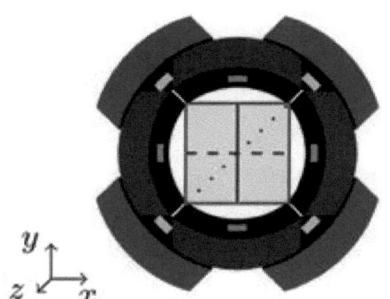 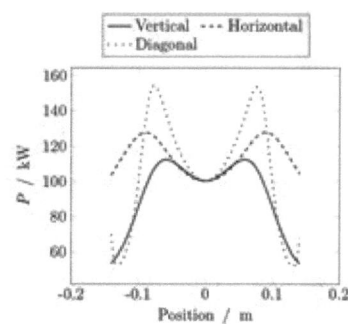

Figure 1: Simulated scanner setup based on the proposed hybrid coil configuration (left) and the corresponding power loss moving an FPP along the main axes and the main diagonal (right).

[1] B. Gleich and J. Weizenecker, "Tomographic imaging using the nonlinear response of magnetic particles", Nature 435, pp. 1214 – 1217, 2005.

[2] I. Schmale, J. Rahmer, B.Gleich, J. Kanzenbach, J. D. Schmidt, C. Bontus, O. Woywode, and J. Borgert, "First phantom in vivo MPI images with an extended field of view", SPIE Medical Imaging 2011: Biomedical Applications in Molecular, Structural, and Functional Imaging, doi: 10.1117/12.877339, 2011.

[3] T. F. Sattel, T. Knopp, S. Biederer, B. Gleich, J. Weizenecker, J. Borgert, and T. M. Buzug, "Single-sided device for magnetic particle imagig", Journal of Physics D: Applied Physics 42(2), pp. 1 – 5, 2009.

[4] T. Knopp, T. F. Sattel, and T. M. Buzug, "Efficient magnetic gradient field generation with arbitrary axial displacement for magnetic particle imaging", IEEE Magnetics Letters 3, pp. 6500104, 2012.

Corresponding Author: C. Kaethner, kaethner@imt.uni-Lübeck.de

P02 MEASUREMENT OF SYSTEM FUNCTIONS WITH EXTENDED FIELD-OF-VIEW

Nils Dennis Nothnagel[1], Javier Sanchez-Gonzalez[1], Aleksi Halkola[2], Jürgen Rahmer[3]

[1]Philips Healthcare Spain, Madrid, Spain
[2]Universität zu Lübeck, Institute of Medical Engineering, Germany
[3]Philips Technologie GmbH, Hamburg, Germany

Magnetic Particle Imaging (MPI) is a new medical imaging technology which obtains dynamic images at high spatial and temporal resolution [1]. Although there are alternative concepts like x-space MPI [2], the common way to obtain an MPI image is by inversion of a system matrix that describes the transformation between spatial distribution of the contrast agent and the measured signal. The system matrix is acquired by moving a small delta-like sample point-by-point through the complete field of view (FoV) and measuring its signal response. A concept has been introduced that disperses a smaller FoV on a larger region by the application of additional homogeneous offset fields, so-called focus fields [3]. Further, it has been experimentally demonstrated that this dispersion can be applied continuously on straight lines, by correction of a static system function measurement [4].

We investigate in this contribution, how this dispersion method behaves on different trajectories than a straight line, like low-frequency Lissajous figures. Further, we measure and simulate a large system function that contains the focus field movement. For the experiments, we use a preclinical MPI scanner at Philips Research, Hamburg, Germany. Drive fields of 16 mT are applied in 2D at 24.5 kHz and 26.4 kHz. Focus fields of up to 24 mT are used with sine frequencies around 15 Hz, which sweep the FoV on low frequency Lissajous trajectories. As a result, we find that the correction method can be applied on more complex trajectories than the linear movement. Scaling the results of the experiments from 2D to 3D, the advantage to time reduction is much more pronounced. Nonetheless, the approach to measure the complete system function can become interesting, when higher focus field frequencies are applied and the calibration procedure time can be reduced, for example by compressed sensing [5] or the use of the System Calibration Unit (SCU) [6].

ACKNOWLEDGMENT
AH and JR acknowledge funding by the German Federal Ministry of Education and Research (BMBF grant FKZ 13N11086).

[1] B. Gleich and J. Weizenecker, «Tomographic imaging using the nonlinear response of magnetic particles,» Nature, vol. 435:7046, p. 1214–1217, 2005.
[2] Saritas, Emine U, Patrick W Goodwill, Laura R Croft, Justin J Konkle, Kuan Lu, Bo Zheng, and Steven M Conolly. "Magnetic Particle Imaging (MPI) for NMR and MRI Researchers." Journal of Magnetic Resonance (San Diego, Calif.: 1997) 229 (April 2013): 116–126. doi:10.1016/j.jmr.2012.11.029.
[3] B. Gleich et al., „Fast MPI Demonstrator with Enlarged Field of View," Proc. ISMRM, p. 18:218, 2010.
[4] J. Rahmer et al., «Fast Continous Motion of the Field of View in Magnetic Particle Imaging,» IWMPI , 2013.
[5] Knopp, Tobias, and Alexander Weber. "Sparse Reconstruction of the Magnetic Particle Imaging System Matrix." IEEE Transactions on Medical Imaging 32, no. 8 (August 2013): 1473–1480. doi:10.1109/TMI.2013.2258029.
[6] Halkola, A., J. Rahmer, B. Gleich, J. Borgert, and T. Buzug. "System Calibration Unit for Magnetic Particle Imaging: System Matrix." In 2013 International Workshop on Magnetic Particle Imaging (IWMPI), 1–1, 2013. doi:10.1109/IWMPI.2013.6528344.

Corresponding Author: N. Nothnagel, Nils.nothnagel@philips.com

P03 PROJECTED TRAVELING WAVE MPI

Patrick Vogel[1,2,3], Martin A. Rückert[1,3], Peter Klauer[1,3], Walter H. Kullmann[3], Peter M. Jakob[1,2], Volker C. Behr[1]

[1]Department of Experimental Physics 5 (Biophysics), University of Würzburg, Germany
[2]Research Center for Magnetic Resonance Bavaria e.V. (MRB), Würzburg, Germany
[3]Institute of Medical Engineering, University of Applied Sciences, Würzburg-Schweinfurt, Germany

The traveling wave approach is an alternative magnetic particle imaging (MPI [1]) scanner design for a fast determination of the distribution of superparamagnetic iron-oxide nanoparticles in 3D [2]. It uses a dynamic linear gradient array (dLGA) for generating and moving a field free point (FFP) linearly along the symmetry axis (z-axis). With additional perpendicular saddle coils the FFP can be moved arbitrarily through the 3D volume (fig. 1a). One issue of the initially presented line-scanning mode (LSM) for scanning a 3D sample is the bad resolution in the x- and y-direction. To improve the resolution at least in one direction (x-direction) the slice-scanning mode (SSM) was proposed [3]. However, the resolution in the y-direction is still not optimal (fig. 1c left).

To overcome this problem the scanning-slice is not moved step by step along the y-axis anymore, but is gradually rotated about the z-axis at defined angles to scan a sequence of radial slices (fig. 1b). Because of the bad resolution perpendicular to the two excitation frequencies of one scanning-slice, the received data can be seen as a projection through the 3D volume at the specific angle.

For the reconstruction of the 3D volume in a first step all slices are deconvolved using Wiener filter and a suitable point spread function (PSF). In a second step the deconvolved projections are placed at their respective angle in a 3D array for calculating in a final step the whole 3D dataset using a Radon transformation.

Using the projected TWMPI approach gives the possibility to overcome the resolution issue using the slice-scanning mode in a TWMPI scanner. In figure 1c the results of the resolution improvement can be seen. Using the common slice-scanning mode the resolution in the y-axis is very bad (fig. 1c left), but using the projected SSM approach the resolution in the x- and y-direction is comparable (fig 1c right).

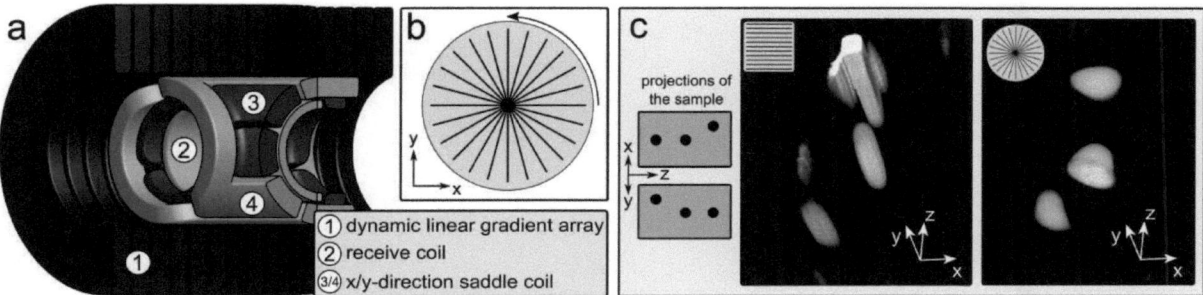

Fig. 1 (a) Sketch of the TWMPI scanner: (1) dynamic linear gradient array (dLGA) for generating and moving the field free point in z-direction, (2) receive coil, (3)/(4) perpendicular saddle coil system for the x- and y-deflection. **(b)** Schematic of radial slice-scanning. **(c)** Improvement of the resolution in the y-direction: on the **left** image the common slice-scanning mode and on the **right** image the radial slice-scanning mode of the same sample.

Corresponding Author: P. Vogel, Patrick.Vogel@physik.uni-Würzburg.de

[1] B. Gleich, and J. Weizenecker, "Tomographic imaging using the nonlinear response of magnetic particles", Nature 435, 1214-1217, Jun. 2005.

[2] P. Vogel et al. „Traveling Wave Magnetic Particle Imaging", IEEE TMI, 2013, Doi: 10.1109/TMI.2013.2285472.

[3] P. Vogel et al."Slicing Frequency Mixed Traveling Wave for 3D Magnetic Particle Imaging", Proc. IWMPI, p. 231f., Lübeck, Germany, 2012 (Springer Proceedings in Physics 140, Magnetic Particle Imaging, 231f., Springer, 2012).

Corresponding Author: P. Vogel, Patrick.Vogel@physik.uni-Würzburg.de

P04 SUPERSPEED TRAVELING WAVE MPI

Patrick Vogel[1,2,3], Martin A. Rückert[1,3], Peter Klauer[1,3], Walter H. Kullmann[3],
Peter M. Jakob[1,2], Volker C. Behr[1]

[1]*Department of Experimental Physics 5 (Biophysics), University of Würzburg, Germany*
[2]*Research Center for Magnetic Resonance Bavaria e.V. (MRB), Würzburg, Germany*
[3]*Institute of Medical Engineering, University of Applied Sciences Würzburg-Schweinfurt, Germany*

The traveling wave magnetic particle imaging (TWMPI) scanner [1] is a progression of the common MPI approach [2]. It uses a dynamic linear gradient array (dLGA) for generating and moving a field free point (FFP) linearly along the z-axis. With additional perpendicular saddle coils the FFP can be moved arbitrarily through a 3D volume. Using the slice-scanning mode (SSM) a 3D volume can be scanned step by step by moving the scanning-slice gradually along the third axis [3].

The scanning time for one slice depends only on the main frequency f_1 driving the dLGA. The secondary excitation frequency f_2 of the SSM is much higher and can generate with each additional period a more densely sampled SSM image, because of the odd relation of the two excitation frequencies. For e.g. a frequency f_1=1 kHz the scanning time for one slice is $t_{slice}=1/2 \cdot 1/f_1$=500 µs (up to 2000 frames per second). The factor ½ stems from the fact, that the dLGA generates two FFPs in one period. Thus, every half period a whole image can be acquired.

In a first test a freely moveable square µ-metal platelet with a side length of 1 mm is scanned with a whole scan time of 20 ms. The result is an image with 250 x 250 pixel and averages. The position of the µ-metal cannot be determined exactly and is smeared in the x-direction (fig. 1 (a)). The reason is the averaging, which means a 40 times passing of a FFP. After a FFP wise reconstruction of the whole dataset, which means that gradually only 25.000 data points are used to create an image instead of using the whole dataset containing 10^6 data points, the exact position of the µ-metal sample can be determined for every FFP pass (every 500 µs) (see fig. 1 (b)). Due to the fewer data points the image resolution of the high speed images decreases to 100 x 100 pixel.

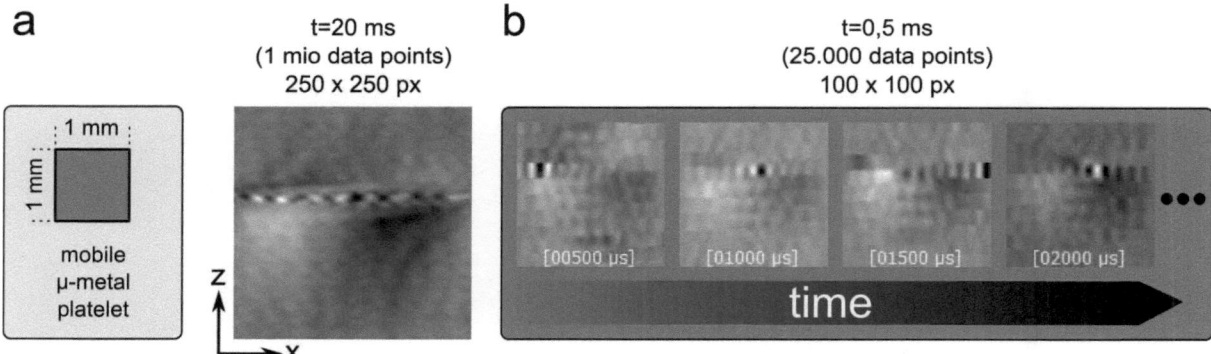

Fig. 1 (a) A freely moveable square µ-metal platelet with 1 mm side length gives a very interesting image after a scan whole time of 20 ms (40 average). No exact position of the sample can be seen. **(b)** The same dataset evaluated for each FFP pass (every 0,5 ms): the exact position of the µ-metal sample can be monitored.

Corresponding Author: P. Vogel, Patrick.Vogel@physik.uni-Würzburg.de

[1] P. Vogel et al. „Traveling Wave Magnetic Particle Imaging", IEEE TMI, 2013, Doi: 10.1109/TMI.2013.2285472.

[2] B. Gleich, and J. Weizenecker, "Tomographic imaging using the nonlinear response of magnetic particles", Nature 435, 1214-1217, Jun. 2005.

[3] P. Vogel et al. "Slicing Frequency Mixed Traveling Wave for 3D Magnetic Particle Imaging", Proc. IWMPI, p. 231f., Lübeck, Germany, 2012 (Springer Proceedings in Physics 140, Magnetic Particle Imaging, 231f., Springer, 2012).

Corresponding Author: P. Vogel, Patrick.Vogel@physik.uni-Würzburg.de

P05 SETUP AND VALIDATION OF AN MPI SIGNAL CHAIN FOR A DRIVE FIELD FREQUENCY OF 150 KHZ

T. F. Sattel[1], O. Woywode[1], J. Weizenecker[2], J. Rahmer[3], B. Gleich[3], J. Borgert[3]

[1]Phillips Medical Systems DMC GmbH, Hamburg, Germany
[2]University of Applied Sciences Karlsruhe, Germany
[3]Philips Technologie GmbH Innovative Technologies, Research Laboratories, Hamburg, Germany

In this contribution, an imaging system is considered, which is part of an activity to test the feasibility of whole-body MPI. Recent studies on nerve stimulation in humans indicate that drive field amplitudes have to be limited to lower values compared to pre-clinical MPI, but that stimulation thresholds increase by moving to frequencies above 100 kHz. Consequently, the three drive field frequencies are set around 150 kHz. To date, available MPI systems usually apply drive fields at frequencies ranging from 1 to 25 kHz. In this contribution, we will report on the technical feasibility of a signal chain set up for a drive field frequency of 150 kHz.

In the experimental set-up, a combined send-receive approach is realized for one imaging dimension. The drive field coil is connected in series with a tuning capacitor assembly (TCA) and an inductive coupling network (ICN). The TCA is tuned such, that the circuit is in resonance at drive field frequency, while the absolute value of the impedance is matched by the ICN configuration. The receive signal is tapped at the TCA. To ensure good drive field signal quality, the power amplifier is connected via a band pass filter to the ICN. To allow for sufficient amplification of the received particle signal, it passes an additional band stop filter before entering the low noise amplifier (LNA).

The signal-to-noise ratio benefits from the drive field frequency shift, since the law of induction implies higher receive sensitivities at higher frequencies. Moreover, the frequency range of the receive signal is well above the noise corner frequency, where the 1/f-noise drops below the flat thermal noise floor. On the other hand, fewer harmonic frequency components are available for image reconstruction when keeping the receive signal bandwidth the same. This matches the fact that also fewer harmonics are generated due to the reduction in drive field amplitude from about 20 mT for preclinical systems to below 10 mT as required by nerve stimulation thresholds.

To validate the function of the implemented MPI signal chain, measurements are performed using Resovist® as nanoparticle tracer material. Furthermore, a permanent magnet configuration is used to generate a selection field gradient that enables low resolution imaging tests. Future plans include the adaption and extension of the set-up to a multi-channel send-receive system with an adjustable gradient field to allow for fast 3-dimensional imaging.

ACKNOWLEDGMENT
This work was supported by the German Federal Ministry of Education and Research (BMBF grant FKZ 13N11086).

Corresponding Author: T. F. Sattel, timo.frederik.sattel@philips.com

P06   TOWARDS A HOLISTIC MPI SIGNAL DETECTION USING A FIELD CANCELATION LOCAL RECEIVE COIL TOPOLOGY

Volkmar Schulz[1,3], Max Mahlke[3], Simon Hubertus[1], Fabian Kiessling[2], Marcel Straub[1]

[1]*Physics of Molecular Imaging Systems, ExMI, RWTH Aachen University, Germany*
[2]*Experimental Molecular Imaging (ExMI), RWTH Aachen University, Germany*
[3]*Philips Research Europe, Aachen, Germany*

MPI is known to be a fast, sensitive imaging modality to measure the distribution of magnetic nanoparticles (MNPs) with high spatial resolution. The first system already offered a spatial resolution in the order of 1 mm and a high temporal resolution with nearly 50 three-dimensional volumes/s [1]. These outstanding system characteristics may make MPI an ideal modality for applications like cell tracking or perfusion imaging.

Beside the optimization of the MNPs, a lot of research is centered on improving the sensitivity and efficiency by proposing new drive-field and focus-field coil topologies, like the field-free-line coils, elliptical coils, or traveling wave coils [2-4]. In combination with harmonic-space MPI the receive chain often contains a high order and low-loss band-stop filter (BSF) to suppress the drive field signal component in the receive signal to avoid saturation of the amplifier or the analog-to-digital conversion. As a side effect the frequency component of the MNP signal at the drive field frequency, which is according to the Langevin theory the largest harmonic component, is automatically absorbed [4]. In [5] different concepts have been proposed which are using signal cancelation based on additional drive-field coil configurations, also in combination with additional filtering.

In difference to [5], this paper will investigate the concept of field cancelation (FC) based on a dedicated receive-coil (RC) design for an existing mouse MPI system from [1] without modifying the drive-field coils. The proposed FC-RC design aims at improving MPI on the following aspects:

Significant reduction of the drive-field signal in the receive chain without absorbing MNP signal components

Reduction of interfering signal pickup from the scanner environment

Enable the holistic signal detection of the MNP response including the excitation frequencies from the drive field coils

The FC-RC L_m consists of a centralized rectangular, bent surface coil L_s with a high sensitivity for the MNP response at the coil's iso-center and an additional symmetrical receive coil pair L_c, as depicted in Fig. a) and b). In order to investigate different RC realizations only half of the cylindrical coil carrier has been used. The linear extension e of the compensation coil L_c was chosen to minimize the mutual inductance M_{md} between drive field coil L_d and the receive coil L_m. Fig c) shows the logarithm of the normalized inductive coupling M_{md} as a function of compensation coil extension e. A clear minimum is indicating the best choice for which both fields (magnetic fields of the drive-field coil and receive coil) are almost orthogonal. Intrinsically the cross coupling between the proposed receive coil and the other two drive fields should be minor. In order to compensate for the remaining coupling of the drive field coils, the signals of the individual compensating coils are measured as well and considered for precise drive field cancelation.

Corresponding Author: V. Schulz, schulz@pmi.rwth-aachen.de

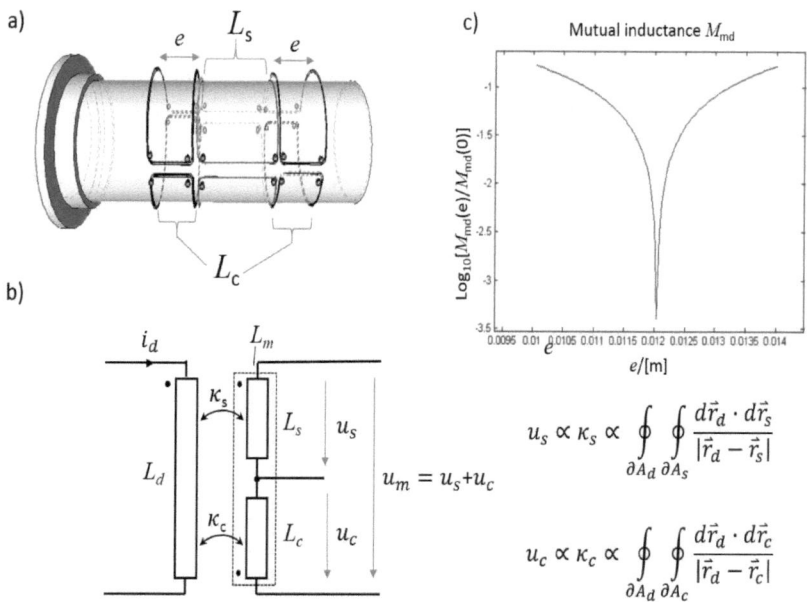

Fig.: a) Upper and lower half cylindrical surface receive coil topology consisting of the MPI-signal-sensing coil (L_s) and compensation coils (L_c), b) schematic coupling of the drive field and one receive coil channel, c) mutual inductive coupling coefficient M_{md} as a function of linear extension e calculated using thin-wire approximations.

In such a way, the new FC-RC design aims at the holistic detection of the response of the magnetic nanoparticles including components at the drive field frequencies supporting harmonic-space and x-space MPI. Therefore, the FC-RC approach has the potential to increase the signal-to-noise ratio (SNR) of the entire MPI acquisition.

Acknowledgement:
The authors would like to thank Philips for their financial support and for providing us with the mouse MPI system from [1].

[1] Weizenecker, J., Gleich, B., Rahmer, J., Dahnke, H., & Borgert, J. (2009). Three-dimensional real-time in vivo magnetic particle imaging. Physics in medicine and biology, 54(5), L1–L10. doi:10.1088/0031-9155/54/5/L01
[2] Konkle, J. J., Goodwill, P. W., Carrasco-Zevallos, O. M., and Conolly, S. M. (2013). Projection reconstruction magnetic particle imaging. IEEE transactions on medical imaging, 32(2), 338–47. doi:10.1109/TMI.2012.2227121
[3] Kaethner, C., Gräfe, K., Gruettner, M., and Buzug, T. M. (2013). Approximated Elliptical Coils In Magnetic Particle Imaging. International Workshop on MPI (Vol. 265, p. 11090).
[4] Vogel, P., Rückert, M. A., Kullmann, W. H., Jakob, P. M., and Behr, V. C. (2013). Slice Scanning Mode For Traveling Wave MPI. In International Workshop on MPI (Vol. 435, p. 796510).
[5] Graeser, M., Knopp, T., Gruettner, M., Sattel, T. F., Bringout, G., Tenner, W., and Buzug, T. M. (2013). Cancellation Techniques for MPI. International Workshop on MPI (Vol. 435, p. 7046).

Corresponding Author: V. Schulz, schulz@pmi.rwth-aachen.de

P07 EXPERIMENTAL DEMONSTRATION OF MULTICHANNEL MAGNETIC PARTICLE IMAGING FOR IMPROVED RESOLUTION

Kuan Lu[1], Patrick Goodwill[1], Steven Conolly[1,2]

[1]Department of Bioengineering, University of California, Berkeley, USA
[2]Department of Electrical Engineering and Computer Science, Berkeley, USA

Introduction: Magnetic particle imaging (MPI) is a promising imaging technique for a great number of clinical and scientific applications ranging from angiography to stem cell tracking. From theory [1-2], spatial resolution in MPI is determined by the strength of the magnetic field gradients as well as the behavior of the nanoparticle contrast agents. Current MPI scanners have a native resolution at the millimeter-scale, which makes small animal and vascular imaging applications difficult. Furthermore, MPI resolution, as with other techniques, is not natively isotropic in all directions. For example, using a one-dimensional drive field, MPI theory shows that the point-spread function (PSF) takes on an anisotropic two-lobed dumbbell shape. Although image-processing techniques like deconvolution may make the final MPI image more isotropic and spatially resolved, these invariably introduce additional noise and artifacts. A more ideal solution is needed to enable sharp and isotropic imaging for clinical diagnostic use. In this work, we experimentally demonstrate that a composition of orthogonal drive and reception channels can create isotropic, high-resolution images using a 3D MPI scanner.

Methods: **Theory**: The native PSF for any arbitrary drive field pattern can be mathematically decomposed into components collinear to and orthogonal to the drive field directions, which contain respectively excellent and poor spatial resolutions for high anisotropy [3]. Analytically, we prove a simple composition of two scans along two orthogonal drive field directions is enough to achieve isotropic resolution in a 2D image for any arbitrary gradient configuration. **Experiment**: We designed and fabricated two sets of transmit and receive coils along two orthogonal directions as above for a 7 T/m 3D MPI small animal imager. We imaged, along the z and x directions, a 4.5x4.5cm UC imaging phantom constructed from tubing (ID: 0.8 mm) filled with undiluted Micromod Nanomag-MIP nanoparticles (mean core diameter 19 nm, Fig. 1a). The reconstructed images are then co-registered and combined for a final isotropic image.

Results: Figure 1b-c shows reconstructed native images of a UC phantom for scans along the z and x directions, respectively. The experimental images are in good agreement with simulation and our theory in that the resolution is optimized along the scanning direction, which could lead to misdiagnosis. For example, the x-direction image does not capture the bottom of the U-shape in either the simulation or the experiment. However, after combining two native images by averaging the coil sensitivity-weighted reconstructions, which is a linear operation with no noise gain, we can overcome the anisotropic signal loss for improved resolution.

Corresponding Author: K. Lu, luckylukuan@berkeley.edu

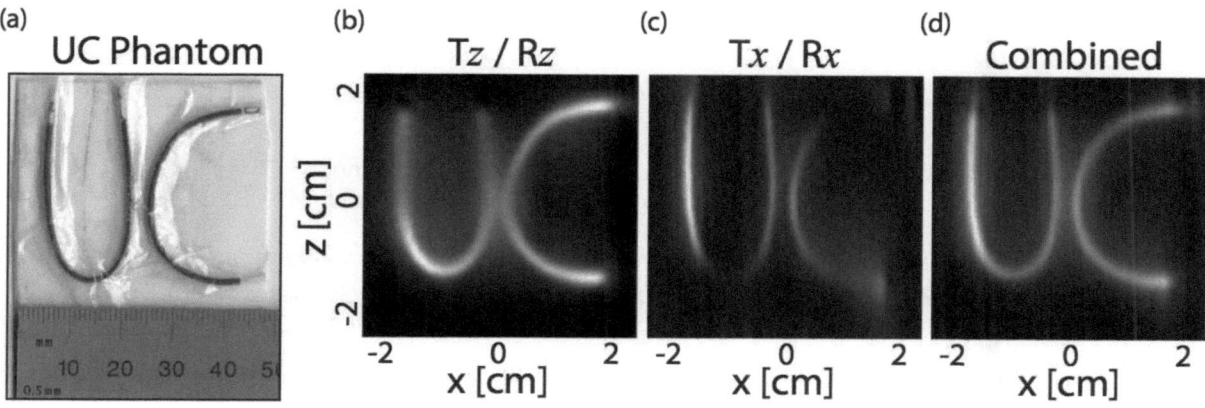

Figure 1 Experimental demonstration of resolution improvement by combining two orthogonal excitation scans. (a) UC phantom injected with Micromod 19nm nanoparticles. (b-c) Native images acquired on 7 T/m scanner by transmitting and receiving in z and x direction, respectively. Image acquisition: 5x4x6cm FOV (along xyz directions), 2 min scan time. (d) Receiver sensitivity-weighted composite images achieve isotropic resolution.

Discussion: In-plane isotropy is of extreme importance to clinical imaging by enabling precise and specific localization of disease, particularly for angiographic applications. In this work, we present a method to achieve isotropic resolution for x-space MPI through combining multiple orthogonal scans. Moreover, we experimentally demonstrate its effectiveness on a small-animal MPI scanner for the first time.

[1] J. Rahmer, J. Weizenecker, B. Gleich, and J. Borgert. BMC Med. Imaging, vol. 9, no. 1, p. 4, 2009.

[2] P Goodwill and S Conolly. IEEE transactions on medical imaging, (c), March 2011

[3] K Lu, B Zheng, J Konkle, EU Saritas, P Goodwill, and S Conolly. IEEE Proceedings on IWMPI 2013, Berkeley, 2013

Corresponding Author: K. Lu, luckylukuan@berkeley.edu

P08 ASYMMETRIC SCANNER DESIGN FOR UNLIMITED PATIENT ACCESS IN MAGNETIC PARTICLE IMAGING

Christian Kaethner[1], Ksenija Gräfe[1], Mandy Ahlborg[1], Gael Bringout[1], Timo F. Sattel[2], Thorsten M. Buzug[1]

[1]Institute of Medical Engineering, Universität zu Lübeck, Germany
[2]Philips Medical Systems DMC GmbH, Hamburg, Germany

Tomographic imaging is an essential part of medical diagnostics today. In addition to clinically established methods, there are several new methods that increase the imaging possibilities and could improve the daily medical routine. Magnetic Particle Imaging (MPI) is one of these new upcoming imaging techniques [1]. This modality being able to acquire quantitative image information of magnetic tracer material using electromagnetic fields shows great characteristics considering spatial resolution, acquisition time, and sensitivity. Due to these properties the attention on MPI grows permanently and makes it an interesting imaging technique, especially for diagnosis or surgical interventions. To realize such interventions, an unlimited patient access from all sides of the patient table for the surgeon is mandatory. Differing from the conventional scanner design in MPI, a circular shaped asymmetric design introduced as single-sided MPI scanner has been proposed, recently [2]. All field generating and data acquiring components are arranged on one side of the patient. This allows designing a patient table integrated scanner solution. In addition to a good patient access, a large field of view (FOV) is required for such interventional scenarios [3,4]. Due to the fact that the recently proposed single-sided MPI scanner is based on circular electromagnetic coils, the width of an adapted patient table would strongly limit the patient access if the scannable FOV is chosen to be sufficiently large. An idea to combine a good patient access with a large FOV is to adapt the outer shape of the electromagnetic coils to the geometry of the patient table (see Figure 1).

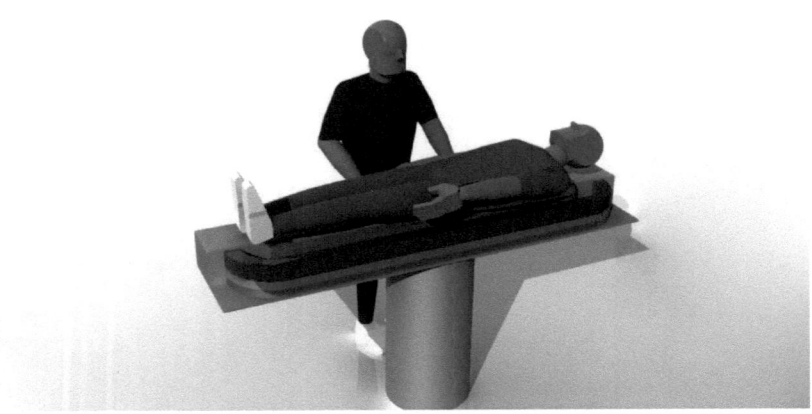

Figure 1: Visualization of the idea to integrate coils into a patient table.

Based on this, first experiments with elliptical coils and approximated elliptical coils were performed recently with promising results for magnetic field properties [5]. Consequently, a suitable asymmetric coil arrangement should be designed that combines the advantages of the circular shaped single-sided device with the generation of a larger FOV. In this contribution, a design study simulating an approximated elliptical single-sided scanner is performed, whereas the focus is on the analysis of the magnetic field strength, the gradient strength, resulting trajectories, and the reconstructed images.

Corresponding Author: C. Kaethner, kaethner@imt.uni-Lübeck.de

These results are compared to the circular single-sided device with comparable gradient strength in the FFP. An interesting point is that the aspect ratio of such an approximated elliptical coil arrangement is an important parameter considering the gradient strength in x, y, and z direction. It can be shown that an enlargement of the trajectory results in promising reconstructed images.

[1] B. Gleich and J. Weizenecker, "Tomographic imaging using the nonlinear response of magnetic particles", Nature 435, pp. 1214 – 1217, 2005.

[2] T. F. Sattel, T. Knopp, S. Biederer, B. Gleich, J. Weizenecker, J. Borgert, and T. M. Buzug, "Single-sided device for magnetic particle imagig", Journal of Physics D: Applied Physics 42(2), pp. 1 – 5, 2009.

[3] J. Haegele, J. Rahmer, B. Gleich, J. Borgert, H. Wojtczyk, N. Panagiotopolos, T. M. Buzug, J. Barkhausen, and F. M. Vogt, "Magnetic particle imaging: visualization of instruments for cardiovascular intervention", Radiology 265(3), pp. 933 – 938, 2012.

[4] J. Haegele, S. Biederer, H. Wojtczyk, M. Graeser, T. Knopp, T. M. Buzug, J. Barkhausen, and F. M. Vogt, "Toward cardiovascular interventions guided by magnetic particle imaging: first instrument characterization", Magnetic Resonance in Medicine 69(6), pp. 1761 – 1767, 2013.

[5] C. Kaethner, M. Ahlborg, K. Gräfe, G. Bringout, T. F. Sattel, and T. M. Buzug, "On the way to a patient table integrated scanner system in magnetic particle imaging", SPIE Medical Imaging 2011: Biomedical Applications in Molecular, Structural, and Functional Imaging, Paper No. 9038-41, 2014.

Corresponding Author: C. Kaethner, kaethner@imt.uni-Lübeck.de

P09 INITIAL RESULTS OF THE FIRST COMMERCIAL PRECLINICAL MPI SCANNER

Jochen Franke[1,2], Ulrich Heinen[1], Alexander Weber[1,2], Nicoleta Baxan[1], Ute Molkentin[1], Sarah Hermann[1], Wolfgang Ruhm[1], Michael Heidenreich[1]

[1]Bruker BioSpin MRI GmbH, Ettlingen, Germany
[2]Institute of Medical Engineering, University of Lübeck, Germany

Magnetic particle imaging (MPI) is a novel tracer-based imaging method allowing the detection of th distribution of superparamagnetic iron oxide (SPIO) nanoparticles in vivo in three dimensions and in real time [1]. Until now, often the main focus of MPI research was MPI technology oriented with many MPI research groups evaluating their own scanner topology with substantially different approaches and features [2,3]. For the important development of real MPI clinical *in vivo* applications, and for the development and *in vivo* comparison of new MPI contrast agents, an easy-to-use and reliable MPI scanner platform needs to be accessible for the MPI research community that fulfills the regulatory requirements for routine *in vivo* applications. In this work, the technical specifications of the first commercially available Preclinical *In Vivo* MPI Scanner will be summarized and its imaging performance will be characterized in terms spatial and temporal resolution and sensitivity limits. A workflow for *in vivo* experiments will be illustrated by an *in vivo* experiment with a rat that was performed under standard *in vivo* laboratory conditions and in which the animal was constantly monitored and kept alive during and after the MPI scan. The workflow for acquisition of anatomical reference MR images during the same session with intermodality transfer of the anesthetized animal and subsequent co-registration of the images is presented.

[1] B. Gleich and J. Weizenecker, Nature, vol. 435, no. 7046, pp.1214–1217, 2005.

[2] Erbe et al., Med Phys. 2011 Sep;38(9):5200-7.

[3] Goodwill et al. Rev Sci Instrum. 2012 Mar;83(3):033708

Corresponding Author: J. Franke, Jochen.Franke@bruker-BioSpin.de

Poster

Imaging Technology and Safety

P10 ULTRA-LOW FIELD MRI TECHNOLOGY USING HIGH-TEMPERATURE SUPERCONDUCTOR SQUID

Junichi Hatta, Shingo Tsunaki, Masaaki Yamamoto, Yoshimi Hatsukade, Saburo Tanaka

Department of Environmental and Life Sciences, Toyohashi University of Technology, Japan

We have developed an ultra-low field (ULF) magnetic resonance imaging (MRI) system utilizing a high-temperature superconductor (HTS) superconducting quantum interference device (SQUID) and a permanent magnet for application of contaminant detection in food [1]. In order to enhance the magnetization of protons and to compensate the shortage of signal-to-noise ratio of the HTS-SQUID based system, the permanent magnet of Halbach layout was employed for the stronger pre-polarizing field B_p. We also introduced a sample transfer apparatus, which can transfer a sample from the permanent magnet to the measuring position under the HTS-SQUID in about 0.5 s. In our system, the ultra-low measurement field B_m generated by a Helmholtz coil is oriented orthogonal to B_p. We considered that the magnetization M of the pre-polarized sample was still nearly parallel to B_p and perpendicular to B_m at the measuring position in a magnetically shielded room (MSR). However, the magnetization M remains in B_p direction only when the magnetic field during the transfer is reduced quickly (sudden passage). When the magnetic field is reduced slowly (adiabatic passage), M follows it and aligns with B_m under the SQUID without any precession occurring [2-3]. Therefore, after the transfer, a π/2 ac pulse is applied to flip M perpendicular to B_m, and then the free induction decays (FID) signal from the sample can be measured by the HTS-SQUID. To improve the FID signal, it is necessary to control the changes in magnetic field strength and direction between the permanent magnet and the measuring position, carefully. We measured 2D MRIs from several samples using the above system. The filtered back projection reconstruction was utilized to obtain the 2D MRIs. Projection number was 12, because the gradient field directions were rotated for 15° step by step to cover 180°. For all projections, SE signals were recorded without averaging. The space resolution is 1.953 Hz/pixel (corresponding to 0.16 cm/pixel), while the field of view (FOV) is 51.2×51.2 mm in area, which correspond to 62.5 Hz in bandwidth, or 32×32 points in pixel. We measured the cucumber sample with a hole using the 2D MRI sequence. The sample is a cucumber of 33 mm in diameter and 8 mm in thickness, which was cut perpendicular to the longitudinal direction. An air hole in raw foods like cucumbers can be a quality problem. The photograph of the cucumber sample with a hole in the center is shown in Figure 1(a). The result of 2D MRI measurement is shown in Figure 1(b). The size of the 2D MRI of the cucumber (about f22 mm) is smaller than the actual sample sizes (about f33 mm) because the sample size is larger than the SQUID's size (about 10 mm square). In the image shown in Figure 1(b), the image intensity at the hole position was clearly low. From this result, it is shown that the hole position can be localized by this technique. As the next challenge, we plan to utilize flux transformer or increase SQUID channel, to expand the SQUID's detection area.

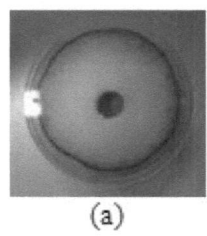
(a)

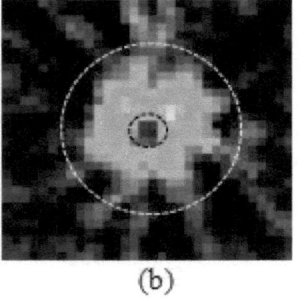
(b)

Fig.1. (a) Cucumber sample with a hole. (b) 2D MRI image of cucumber sample with a hole.

Corresponding Author: J. Hatta, jh004@edu.imc.tut.ac.jp

We also began to investigate another system with a polarizing coil in place of the permanent magnet and the sample transfer apparatus. The liquid nitrogen-cooled polarizing coil utilizing the HTS wire, Di-BSCCO wire produced by Sumitomo Electric Industries, Ltd., produce higher B_p than 100 mT at the sample. The self-shielded polarizing coil would reduce the eddy currents induced in the conductive layers of the MSR when B_p is switched off rapidly. The fast decay time of the field B_p can be applied to the measurements of samples which have a shorter relaxation time T_1 such as biological samples. This system will be applied to acquire images for small animals. The magnetic particle imaging (MPI) signal originates particularly from the administered tracer material which makes an unambiguous assignment to an anatomical region difficult. To overcome this lack of anatomical information, one can superpose the MPI data with anatomical images acquired with e.g. MRI. The small animal ULF-MRI will also be used to acquire reference images for the MPI data. In the near future, we will construct a MRI food contaminant detection system combining with MPI technology.

This work was supported in part by The Knowledge Hub of Aichi, The priority Research Project.

[1] Yoshimi Hatsukade, Shingo Tsunaki, Masaaki Yamamoto, Takayuki Abe, Junichi Hatta, and Saburo Tanaka, "Feasibility study of contaminant detection for food with ULF-NMR/MRI system using HTS-SQUID," Physica C 494, 199 (2013).

[2] B.F. Melton, V.L. Pollak, T.W. Mayes, and B.L. Willis, "Condition for sudden passage in the Earth's-field NMR Technique," J. Magn. Reson. A 117, 164 (1995).

[3] B.F. Melton, and V.L. Pollak, "Condition for adiabatic passage in the Earth's-field NMR Technique," J. Magn. Reson. 158, 15 (2002).

Corresponding Author: J. Hatta, jh004@edu.imc.tut.ac.jp

P11 EXPERIMENTAL EVALUATION OF ITERATIVE RECONSTRUCTION METHOD FOR TIME-CORRELATION MAGNETIC PARTICLE IMAGING

Hiroki Tsuchiya[2], Takumi Homma[1], Syota Shimizu[1], Yasutoshi Ishihara[2]

[1]Graduate School of Science and Technology, Meiji University, Kanagawa, Japan
[2]School of Science and Technology, Meiji University, Kanagawa, Japan

Magnetic particle imaging (MPI) is reconstructed with signals generated from magnetic nanoparticles (MNPs) at the field-free point (FFP) in the field of view (FOV)[1]. However, image blurring and artifacts due to the interference of the magnetization response generated from outside of the FFP region appear when the magnetic field is insufficient to saturate the magnetization of MNPs. Therefore, we have proposed an original reconstruction method as one solution to solve this problem. In our method, the image is reconstructed with time-correlation information between the observed signal from MNPs and the corresponding system function at each FFP[2,3]. However, image blurring and artifacts have not improved enough with this method because the observed signal also indicates high correlation for the system function near the FFP. Last year, we proposed a new iterative image reconstruction method[4]. In this process (Fig1 (a)), (1) the initial reconstructed image is calculated by our previous time-correlation reconstruction method, (2) the differences between the waveforms estimated from each reconstructed image and the observed signals are calculated, (3) the error images are computed on the basis of the correlation with these differences and the corresponding system function at each FFP, and (4) the iterative image is reconstructed by adding the error image to the initial image or the previous iterative image. By repeating a series of such processes, the iterative image is expected to converge to the exact particle distribution, reducing image blurring and artifacts. We have performed some experiments (Fig1 (b), (c), (d)) with our prototype system to confirm the validity of this method. In our experiments, we used a Maxwell pair coil with a 180-mm diameter (space between opposite coils: 50 mm) and a receiver coil with a 35-mm diameter (placed at a position 35 mm from the Maxwell coil's center). A gradient magnetic field of approximately 1.65 T/m was applied in the x direction, and an alternating magnetic field of 20 mT was applied in the same direction. A FOV with a matrix size of 21 × 21 was set to be 30 mm × 30 mm.

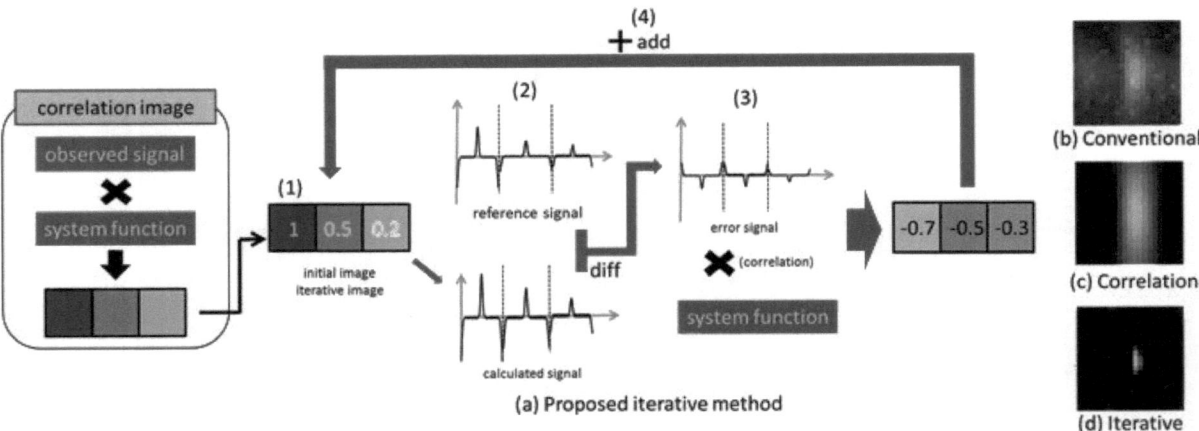

Figure1 Proposed method and results

Corresponding Author: H. Tsuchiya, ee04113@meiji.ac.jp

The proposed method improved image artifacts and blurring up to about 3 times compared to the conventional method. However, the effect of the improvement in image quality was insufficient compared with the results of the past numerical analysis. As one reason for this difference, it is possible that the system function calculated analytically was used in the experiment. In particular, as it is clear that a system function differs from the theoretical value on the boundary of the FOV in our system, a more accurate three-dimensional system function needs to be acquired in the future. Furthermore, a proposal for an algorithm that improves the feedback method with the error image during iterative processing and an appropriate successive approximation is required.

[1] Gleich B, Weizenecker J: Tomographic imaging using the nonlinear response of magnetic particles, Nature 435 (30), pp. 1214 – 1217, 2005.

[2] Ishihara Y, Kuwabara T, Homma T, Nakagawa Y: Correlation-based image reconstruction methods for magnetic particle imaging, IEICE Trans Inf Syst. E95-D (3), pp. 872 – 879, 2012.

[3] Ishihara Y, Homma T, Nohara S, Ito Y: Evaluation of magnetic nanoparticle samples made from ferucarbotran having excellent biocom patibility by time-correlation magnetic particle imaging reconstruction method, BMC Medical Imaging 2013, 13:15, 2013.

[4] Homma T, Shimizu S, Ishihara Y: Reduction of image blurring for time-correlation magnetic particle imaging, IWMPI 2013.

Corresponding Author: H. Tsuchiya, ee04113@meiji.ac.jp

P12 SYSTEM MATRIX RECORDING AND PHANTOM MEASUREMENTS WITH A SINGLE-SIDED MPI SCANNER

Ksenija Gräfe[1], Gael Bringout[1], Matthias Graeser[1], Timo Sattel[2], Thorsten M. Buzug[1]

[1]*Institute of Medical Engineering, University of Lübeck, Germany*
[2]*Phillips Medical Systems DMC GmbH, Hamburg, Germany*

A prototype of a single-sided magnetic particle imaging (MPI) scanner has been presented in 2009 by Sattel et al. [1]. In comparison to other scanner geometries, the single-sided scanner design offers a perfect patient access through its open design. In this work, a set up of an improved oil cooled design is presented. This scanner consists of two concentrically arranged circular coils for the one dimensional (1D) imaging process and an additional D-shaped coil pair, which lies flat under the circular coils, to realize two dimensional (2D) imaging. A direct current of about 55 A is applied to the outer coil and about 65 A to the inner coil. They flow in opposite direction. The superposition of the resulting magnetic fields results in two field free points (FFP), one in front of the scanner and one behind the scanner. For the imaging process, only the FFP in front of the scanner is used. In addition, an alternating current (AC) of 42 A at a frequency of about 25 kHz on the inner coil is applied to move the FFP in axial direction [2]. For 2D imaging, an AC on the D-shaped coil is necessary. At the moment, the 2D part is under construction and it is possible to record a 1D system matrix and 1D phantom measurements.

This paper presents the first test results with the oil cooled scanner device. First, different samples of Resovist® have been tested to find the best sample sizes to record the system matrix and to get an estimation of the resulting penetration depth. As the magnetic field amplitude decrease with the distance to the scanner, the penetration depth and resolution will be limited. A special sample holder for measuring the system matrix has been constructed and a system matrix has been recorded. In the next step, the analysis of the signal to noise ratio (SNR) provides a limit of the achievable resolution. For the reconstruction, only the frequency components with an SNR above 10 have been used and a 1D phantom has been reconstructed (Figure 1).

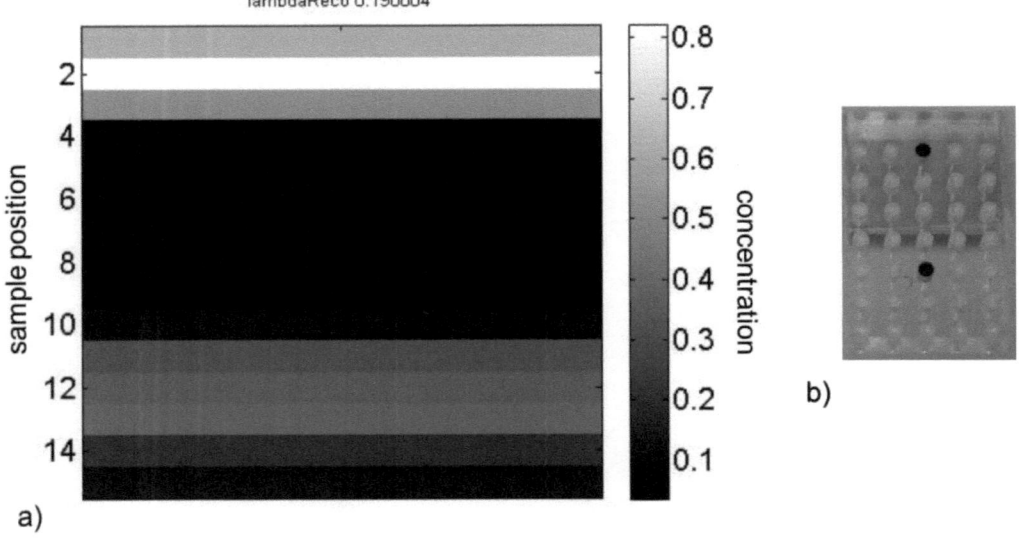

Figure 1: The reconstruction result a) of a phantom b) with two sample points, the first one in a distance of about 4 mm to the scanner and the second one in a distance of about 22 mm.

Corresponding Author: K. Gräfe, graefe@imt.uni-Lübeck.de

Acknowledgements

This project has been supported by the German Federal Ministry of Education and Research (BMBF Grant Number 01EZ0912).

References

[1] T. F. Sattel, T. Knopp, S. Biederer, B. Gleich, J. Weizenecker, J. Borgert and T. M. Buzug, "Single-sided device for magnetic particle imaging", Journal of Physics D: Applied Physics, vol. 42, no. 2, 5 pages, January 2009.

[2] T. F. Sattel, M. Erbe, S. Biederer, T. Knopp, D. Finas, K. Diedrich, K. Lüdtke-Buzug, J. Borgert, T. M. Buzug, "Single-sided magnetic particle imaging device for the sentinel lymph node biopsy scenario", Proc. SPIE 8317, Medical Imaging 2012: Biomedical Applications in Molecular, Structural, and Functional Imaging, 83170S, March 2012.

Corresponding Author: K. Gräfe, graefe@imt.uni-Lübeck.de

P13 CONSTRUCTION OF A MULTI-DIMENSIONAL TRANSMIT FIELD GENERATOR AND RECEIVE COIL SETUP

Matthias Gräser[1], Timo Sattel[2], Thorsten M. Buzug[1]

[1] Institute of Medical Engineering, University of Lübeck, Germany
[2] Phillips Medical Systems DMC GmbH Hamburg, Germany

In most multi-dimensional dynamic magnetic particle imaging devices, several frequencies are used to move the field free point (FFP) or field free line (FFL) through the space [1, 2]. The used fields corresponding to these frequencies are orthogonal and superimposed by the static selection field, which has a different alignment in each spatial position. In spectrometer setups in contrast, only one excitation field and one superimposed offset field are used [3]. Due to relaxation effects and frequency mixing, the measurements of a 1D spectrometer setup are not directly comparable to the measurements of a scanning device.

This work addresses the design and construction of a three dimensional spectrometer setup. Most 1D spectrometers use a solenoid send coil and a dedicated solenoid receive coil to measure the particle response to a well-known magnetic field sequence. This setup must now be supplemented by two additional orthogonal transmit and receive coils. These coils cannot be realized as solenoid coils, thus other approaches have to be developed.

Starting from a current distribution, directed along the tube axis of a cylinder generate a magnetic field inside of its cylindrical surface. Neglecting boundary effects the field gets homogeneous, if the amplitude of the current distribution is sinusoidal dependent on the angle to the tube axis [4, 5]. Such a current distribution cannot be realized, and boundary effects will introduce inhomogeneities. By adapting the continuous current distribution by discrete wires, the position of the wires can be found by minimizing the error of the current distribution integral. Thus an optimal coil shape can be realized that generate a highly homogeneous perpendicular field profile to the solenoid without limiting the bore of the first coil. The third field direction is generated by a similar shaped coil, with slightly larger bore to fit around the other two coils.

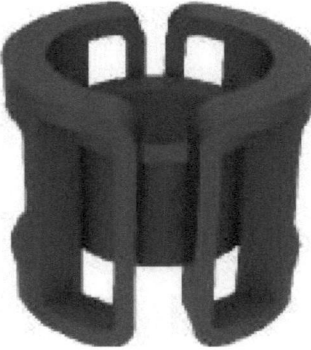

Figure 1 2D-coil setup design with homogeneous cage coil

To receive the particle signal, one has to design a set of receive coils that fits inside the field generation setup. The designed coils resemble the transmit coils in appearance, thus due to the smaller wire cross section, the approximation of the continuous current distribution can be more accurate.

Corresponding Author: M. Gräser, graeser@imt.uni-Lübeck.de

To be able to neglect all coupling effects of such a 3D setup, a cancellation unit is build, with the same geometry of the field generator. Thus, not only couplings of the send coils can be attenuated but also the receive chain and send chain can be magnetically decoupled. Therefore, the transmit filter can be more compact, because disturbing signals like harmonics in the send chain cannot interfere with the receive chain.

With the realized setup, any field sequence in an existing or fictive scanner can be emulated. This allows for predicting image resolution and magnetization relaxation effects, as well as the measurement of the scanner's point spread function that can be used to deconvolute an X-Space reconstructed image.

We acknowledge the Federal Ministry of Education and Research, Germany under grant number 13N11090 as well as the European Union and the State Schleswig-Holstein (Program for the Future-Economy: 122-10-004).

[1] B. Gleich and J. Weizenecker, "Tomographic imagingusing the nonlinear response of magnetic particles," Nature, vol. 435, no. 7046, pp. 1214–1217, 2005.
[2] T. Knopp et. al., "Field-free line formation in a magnetic field," Journal of Physics A: Mathematical and Theoretical., vol. 43, no. 1, p. 9pp, 2010.
[3] S. Biederer et. al., "Magnetization response spectroscopy of superparamagnetic nanoparticles for magnetic particle imaging," Journal of Physics D: Applied Physics, vol. 42, no. 20, p. 7pp, 2009.
[4] T. Sattel et. al., "Experimental setup of receive coils with trans axial sensitivity profiles," in IWMPI, 2013.
[5] D. Lobb, "Properties of some useful two-dimensional magnetic fields," Nuclear Instruments and Methods, vol. 64, no. 3, pp. 251–267, 168.

Corresponding Author: M. Gräser, graeser@imt.uni-Lübeck.de

P14 CHALLENGES OF STABLE MRI DATA ACQUISITION USING THE PRECLINICAL MPI-MRI HYBRID SYSTEM

Jochen Franke[1,2], Sascha Köhler[1], Franek Hennel[1], Alexander Weber[1,2], Ulrich Heinen[1], Wolfgang Ruhm[1], Michael Heidenreich[1], Thorsten M. Buzug[2]

[1]*Bruker BioSpin MRI GmbH, Ettlingen, Germany*
[2]*Institute of Medical Engineering, University of Lübeck, Germany*

Magnetic particle imaging (MPI) is a novel tracer-based imaging method allowing detection of the distribution of superparamagnetic iron oxide (SPIO) nanoparticles *in vivo* in three dimensions and in real time [1]. However, MPI lacks of the detection of morphological information in order to unambiguously assign the spatial SPIO distribution to the actual organ structures. Therefore, merging the quantitative information of the spatial distribution of the contrast agent acquired with a MPI scanner with the morphological data e.g. acquired with a MRI scanner has been shown to be a promising approach. So far, this has been accomplished by using two independent scanners [2]. Image fusion with high spatial and temporal confidence necessitates a hybrid scanner in which no or at most an easy object transfer and no anesthesia interruption of the animal is required. First hybrid scanner approaches have been presented in 2013. The implementation of stable MR imaging on hybrid scanners realized by resistive magnet designs can be challenging due to magnet and power supply instabilities. In this work, we present significant improvements achieved by adaption of the current control loop parameters of the magnet power supply as well as stabilized cooling of the resistive magnet. Latter improvement is essential as a temperature fluctuation in cooling media results in fluctuation of the median magnet temperature causing directly B_0 field drifts. This sensitive temperature effect is well known from the past of using resistive magnets in MRI and cannot be fully eliminated by means a justifiable effort. In this work we present an additional approach detecting and correcting for residual field instabilities by using newly implemented MRI sequences comprising MRI navigators. Here, the MRI navigator signal is analyzed in regard of frequency and phase information, while a real-time processor integrates this information online into the reference frequency of the scanner and thereby into the data flow to automatically correct for the actual B_0 field offset. Two MRI sequences have been adapted to allow for MRI navigator signal detection. Here, the navigator signal is derived from the slice-gradient refocused free-induced-decay (FID) formed by a slice excitation pulse. The dedicated Spin Echo sequence uses the refocused excitation pulse FID of the actual imaging slice, whereas the dedicated Gradient Echo sequence allows to derive the B_0 field offset information from an additional navigator slice. Combination of both, hardware stabilization and the usage of dedicated MR sequences, allows for stable MRI data acquisition using the Preclinical Hybrid MPI-MRI system without the need for any user interaction. The impact of the current control stabilization and the magnet coolant temperature stabilization will be presented by B_0 field stability tests tracking the magnet coolant temperature simultaneous with FID analysis. Combination of both above mentioned improvements were compared to the initial state using MR phantom data. Here, image quality was evaluated in terms of artifacts and signal-to-noise ratios. In addition, a short review of the hybrid hardware scanner specification description and the state of implementation will be presented.

Acknowledgements: The authors thankfully acknowledge the financial support by the German Federal Ministry of Education and Research, FKZ 13N11088.

[1] B. Gleich and J. Weizenecker, Nature, vol. 435, no. 7046, pp.1214–1217, 2005.
[2] Weizenecker J, Gleich B, Rahmer J, Dahnke H, and Borgert J., Phys. Med. Biol. 54(5):L1-L10. 2009.

Corresponding Author: J. Franke, Jochen.Franke@bruker-BioSpin.de

P15 AUTOMATED DERIVATION OF SUB-VOLUME SYSTEM FUNCTIONS FOR 3D MPI WITH FAST CONTINUOUS FOCUS FIELD VARIATION

J. Rahmer[1], B. Gleich[1], C. Bontus[1], J. Schmidt[1], I. Schmale[1], J. Borgert[1], O. Woywode[2], A. Halkola[3], T. Buzug[3]

[1]Philips Technologie GmbH Innovative Technologies, Research Laboratories, Hamburg, Germany
[2]Philips Medical Systems DMC GmbH, Hamburg, Germany
[3]Institute of Medical Engineering, University of Lübeck, Germany

For fast volumetric MPI, orthogonal drive fields are used to move the field-free-point on a 3D trajectory. Image reconstruction then requires the knowledge of a system function (SF) that relates signal to spatial position. The SF is typically determined in a calibration scan over the volume covered by the drive field trajectory. For increased spatial coverage, strong offset fields, called focus fields (FFs) [1, 2], are applied. The increase in imaging volume, however, can lead to prohibitively long calibration scan times. Due to the local nature of MPI encoding, it is possible to split the large volume into sub-volumes, which correspond to the volumes encoded during a single repetition of the drive field sequence. The SFs can be derived for each of these sub-volumes from a single "static" SF determined on the small volume covered by the drive field excitation alone [3]. This is possible, even when the FF changes continuously during the drive field sequence. For derivation of the corresponding "dynamic" SFs, one has to take into account the FF-induced translation of the field-of-view (FOV) and apply a time-domain correction to the static SF [3]. Since the FOV motion is influenced by dynamic eddy current effects, it cannot be determined by the currents applied to the FF coils alone. Eddy current effects have not been taken into account in previous implementations, but for high-resolution imaging, it is mandatory to know the exact FF evolution. To this end, a 3D field sensor is placed in the scanner bore and the FF evolution is measured for the FF sequence used for large-volume object scanning. From the measured FF values, the time-dependent FOV translation is determined via the known selection field gradient and is used for the time-domain derivation of the required dynamic SFs from the measured static SF. In this way, dynamic SFs for all FOV motion states occurring during the FF sequence are generated and the image can be reconstructed over the total imaging volume. It will be shown that this approach also works for rather complex FF trajectories, allowing rapid spatial coverage of large volumes by continuously shifting the FOV along a path that is designed to cover the object to be imaged.

ACKNOWLEDGMENT

This work is supported by the German Federal Ministry of Education and Research (BMBF grant FKZ 13N11086).

[1] B. Gleich et al., "Fast MPI Demonstrator with Enlarged Field of View.", Proc. ISMRM, 18:218, 2010.

[2] P.W. Goodwill and S. M. Conolly, "Multidimensional X-space Magnetic Particle Imaging.", IEEE TMI 30, 9 (2011): 1581–1590.

[3] J. Rahmer et al., "Fast Continuous Motion of the Field of View in Magnetic Particle Imaging.", IEEE Proc. IWMPI 2013.

Corresponding Author: J. Rahmer, Jürgen.rahmer@philips.com

P16 SHIELDED DRIVE COILS FOR A RABBIT SIZED FFL SCANNER

Gael Bringout, Mandy Ahlborg, Matthias Gräser, Christian Kaethner, Jan Stelzner, Wiebke Tenner, Hanne Wojtczyk, Thorsten M. Buzug

Institute of Medical Engineering, University of Lübeck, Germany

In magnetic particle imaging scanners, two main types of field free space are used, namely the point and the line. When the field topologies are of little influence for the first of them, the line properties strongly depend on the field topology. In fact, all generated fields inside the scanner will influence at different degrees the line shape. Moreover, MPI scanners use low inductivities\high voltage coils to generate the drive fields and high inductivity\low voltage coils to generate the selection fields. Therefore, even a small coupling between the drive coils and the selection coils would results in high voltage peak on the selection coils, which is too constraining to be absorbed by the coils. Instead, it would be preferred to shield the selection coils against the high frequency fields. Doing so leads to the generation of eddy current in the shield, which will in returns change the topology of the drive fields.

We designed the drive coils for a rabbit sized FFL scanner using a boundary elements formulation. The induced current in the shield is calculated using the same approach and compared with the results obtained with a commercial finite elements program using an 3D model of the coil. To validate both modeling, the power loss are compared with analytics formula. Finally, the spherical harmonics decomposition of the unshielded coil and the shielded coils are compared.

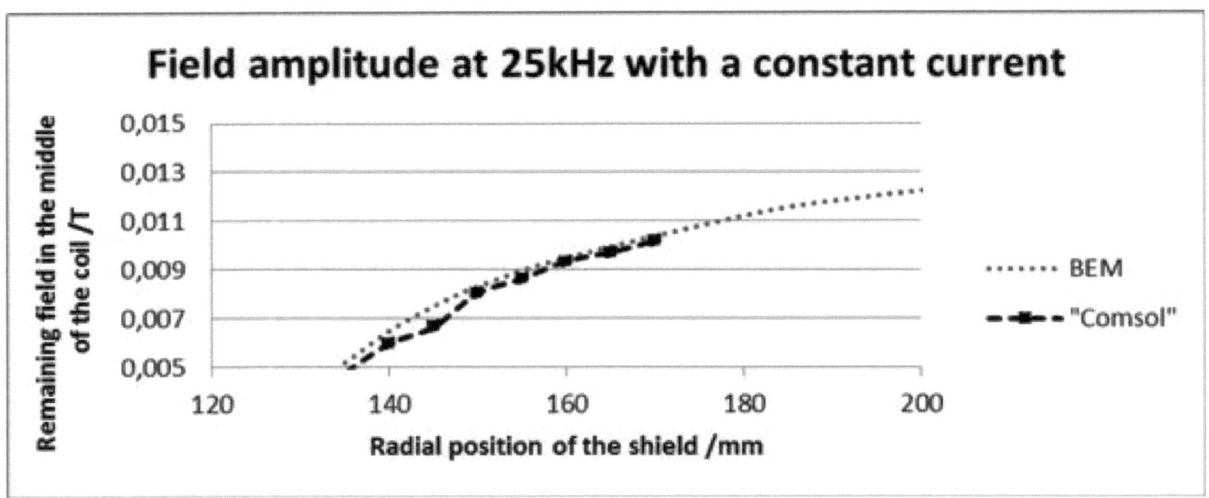

Figure 1: Comparison of the fields in the middle of the coil. Both results are in agreements.

Both methods are able to model the phenomena accordingly to the theory. But, when Comsol© require a mesh with a resolution of the skin depth on the shield (i.e. 0.4 mm in this case), the BEM just need a coarse meshing of the surfaces. The Comsol© calculation required 12 Gb of RAM and 2 hours of calculation per configuration, where the BEM model needed 160Mb of RAM and 286 seconds on the same computer.

The presented methods allowed to correct the efficiency of the coil to take into account the reduction of efficiency of the shielded coil and to plan accordingly the diameter of the shield.

Corresponding Author: G. Bringout, bringout@imt.uni-Lübeck.de

P17 TECHNICAL ASPECTS OF A TWO DIMENSIONAL ROTATABLE FIELD FREE LINE IMAGER FOR MAGNETIC PARTICLE IMAGING

Matthias Weber, Klaas Bente, Matthias Gräser, Mandy Ahlborg, Anselm v. Gladiss, Ksenija Gräfe, Gael Bringout, Marlitt Erbe, Timo F. Sattel, Thorsten M. Buzug

Institute of Medical Engineering, University of Lübeck, Germany

A promising and alternative spatial encoding scheme for Magnetic Particle Imaging (MPI) is based on a field-free line (FFL) [1]. This facilitates following crucial advantages in comparison to conventional field-free point (FFP) imaging techniques.

It is possible to increase the sensitivity by one order of magnitude, thus smaller particle concentrations become visible. Furthermore, due to the projective characteristics of the FFL trajectory, image reconstruction enhances significantly: well-known Radon-based reconstruction algorithms speed-up this process and no system matrix has to be measured and inverted. Nevertheless, two-dimensional FFL-imaging with a rotated FFL has not been realized to the present-day, since high power loss and complex scanner design limited practical implementation.

In this work we present the first two-dimensional FFL images with a rotated FFL and describe the setup. Our system consists of three main parts: the field-generating array, the signal-generating path and the receiving path. In the center the field generating array frames the scanner environment. It is based on custom-built curved rectangular coils embedded in a gantry design featuring an air-cooling system [2]. Selection field coils combined with two permanent magnets generate and rotate the FFL and determine spatial encoding. Additionally, drive field coils allow shifting of the FFL to excite the particles. The whole setup is positioned in a shielding room. Furthermore, the second part adds the signal-generating component to the system. It can be split up into two units: excitation path and spatial encoding path. The signal for the drive field coils is filtered with a 3rd order Butterworth-Filter when it enters the shielding room and is impedance matched with a resonant circuit. Unipolar direct current sources provide the necessary currents for the selection field. Purchased low pass cabin filters avoid interfering signals in the shielding room. Due to the unipolar characteristic a switch system is installed behind it to ensure a complete FFL rotation and has to be operated manually. Furthermore, a fundamental frequency matched resonant circuit protects the direct current sources from any coupled signals between drive and selection field coils. Both paths are fully shielded with copper. The third part completes the system and the receive path. A fitted receive coil array is used to measure the particle signal, which is first filtered in a 4th order Butterworth-Filter to get rid of the fundamental frequency, and afterwards low noise amplified. We send the signal via a differential path to the computer for further signal processing steps. Signal generation and acquisition is facilitated with a self-implemented C++ script generating the raw data. Afterwards, the raw data is processed with MATLAB. Here, signal reconstruction is based on the x-space theory to visualize the reconstructed particle distribution.

[1] J. Weizenecker, B. Gleich, and J. Borgert. Magnetic particle imaging using a field free line. J Appl Phys, 41(10):105009, 2008

[2] M. Erbe, M. Weber, T. F. Sattel and T. M. Buzug. Experimental Validation of an Assembly of Optimized Curved Rectangular Coils for the use in Dynamic Field Free Line Magnetic Particle Imaging. Current Medical Imaging Reviews, 9(2):89-95, 2013

Corresponding Author: M. Weber, weber@imt-uni-Lübeck.de

P18 MAGNETIC PARTICLE IMAGING WITH HIGH-T_c BASED SQUID SENSOR

Hong-Chang Yang[1], Herng-Er Horng[2], Shu-Hsien Liao[2], Jen-Je Chieh[2]

[1]Department of Electro-optical Engineering, Kun Shan University, Tainan, Taiwan
[2]Institute of Electro-optical Science and Technology, National Taiwan Normal University, Taipei, Taiwan

Magnetic particle imaging (MPI) is a new method of medical imaging which performs a direct measurement of the magnetization of magnetic nanoparticles. In this paper, we set up a 2-dimensional magnetic nanoparticle imaging system with high-T_c SQUID sensor. For imaging the magnetic nanoparticle, a pair of magnets, ac excitation coil and dc bias coil are employed to generate a strong gradient filed, excitation field, and bias magnetic field respectively. A pair of pick coils designed as gradiometer is used for detecting the AC magnetization signal of magnetic particles and coupling to the high-T_c SQUID magnetometer via flux coupling method. The minimum volume and concentration of magnetic fluid are identified. The 2-D imaging of phantom are demonstrated by using our high-T_c SQUID based magnetic particle imaging system.

Corresponding Author: H.-C. Yang, hcyang@phys.ntu.edu.tw

P19 MPI BASED HYBRID DESIGN FOR ACTUATION AND MONITORING OF MAGNETIC NANOPARTICLES FOR TARGETED DRUG DELIVERY

Ammar Mahmood[1], Mohammad Dadkhah[2], Jungwon Yoon[3]

[1,2]*Robots & Intelligent Systems Lab, Gyeongsang National University, Jinju, South Korea*
[3] *Department of Mechanical Engineering, Gyeongsang National University, Jinju, South Korea*

Targeted drug delivery is an efficient technique to deliver the drug molecules to the specific tissues in the human body by attaching them to magnetic nanoparticles (MNPs). Electromagnetic actuation systems are the most efficient for applying an adequate force to steer the MNPs in the blood vessels. [1] A monitoring system for the position feedback of the MNPs based on the magnet particle imaging concept is proposed in this paper. A 3D actuation system have been designed and simulated for the actuation of MNPs in [2]. The aim of the proposed system is to investigate the feasibilty of combining the actuation system with magnetic particle imaging (MPI) system using numerical simulations and optimizing hardware constraints. The MNPs can be steered by applying a magnetic field gradient provided by the actuation system in [2] and monitored by applying the drive and selection fields to the actuation coils using a time division multiplexing scheme. Since the drug is loaded on the magnetic particles, the tracer particles in the MPI can be used as carriers. The challenge in this research is to sequence the actuation signal and the MPI signal to perform both tasks simultaneously. Additional coils i.e receive coils are added to our actuation system in [2] to make it compatible with the MPI system. The actuation signal involves a constant current to the coils to generate a magnetic gradient field. The MPI signal cosists of a low frequency sinusoid and a constant current signal superimposed together to move the FFP in the workspace. The receiver coil and the high frequency excitation coil are merged together in a single coil for each axis.(Fig 1) The COMSOL Multiphysics software is used for modeling and simulation of the system. The proposed system will provide simultaneous navigation and tracking for targeted drug delivery of magnetic nanoparticles in compact and efficent ways.

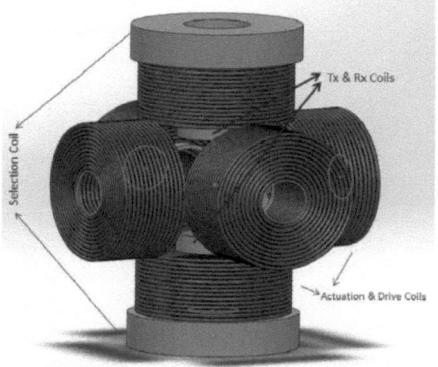

Fig 1. Schematic drawing of the proposed hybrid system showing the additional coils added to our actuation system.

Acknowledgement: This research was supported by the Pioneer Research Centre Program through the National Research Foundation of Korea funded by the Ministry of Education, Science and Technology (NRF 2012-0009524).

[1] Yesin, K. B., Vollmers, K. and Nelson, B. , 'Modeling and control of unthered biomicrorobots in a fluidic environment using electromagnetic fields.' The International Journal of Robotics Research, 25(5–6): 527–536, 2006

[2] Mohammad Dadkhah, Naveen Kumar, Jungwon Yoon, 'Design and Simulation of a 3D Actuation System for Magnetic Nano-Particles Delivery System',6th International Conference, ICIRA 2013, Busan, South Korea, September 25-28, 2013

Corresponding Author: Mahmood, ammarmahmood@live.com

Poster

Modelling, Simulation, Reconstruction & Sequences

P20 COMPARISON OF X-SPACE AND CHEBYSHEV RECONSTRUCTION IN MAGNETIC PARTICLE IMAGING

Mandy Ahlborg[1], Tobias Knopp[2], Thorsten M. Buzug[1]

[1]Institute of Medical Engineering, Universität zu Lübeck, Germany
[2]Thorlabs GmbH, Lübeck, Germany

Image reconstruction in Magnetic Particle Imaging (MPI) remains a challenging topic. So far, the developed approaches (for an overview cf. [1]) are for the most part either inefficient or lack image quality mostly due to the unknown particle characteristics of the used MPI tracer. The first MPI image reconstructions were based on a measured calibration procedure to set up a system matrix including the behavior of a particular tracer in a specific scanner configuration [2]. This approach results in high quality images but is tedious and also far too time consuming for clinical applications. Consequentially, the development of a model-based reconstruction was promoted either by realistic [3] or ideal [4, 5] field assumptions. Assuming optimal conditions concerning particle behavior and field quality it was proven by Rahmer et al. that the 1D MPI system matrix is similar to Chebyshev polynomials and 2D/3D system matrices are related to tensor products of Chebyshev polynomials [4]. Further, the comparison with measured system matrices shows a high resemblance and possibly can form a promising basis for image reconstruction. Whereas the Chebyshev approach is performed in Fourier space a second technique assuming ideal conditions with data processing in time domain has been developed. This approach, established by Goodwill et al., is often referred to as x-space reconstruction [4] and is convincing regarding the compactness and speed of the image reconstruction. In x-space MPI the time dependent received signal is directly used, compensated for the field free point velocity and gridded in order to map it to the corresponding spatial position in the field of view. The reconstructed image is called native image. Since the convolution kernel depends on the orientation of the field free point it is moved on a linear trajectory instead of a high frequency sinusoidal trajectory used for the other imaging approaches in MPI. Image reconstruction results of the native image can be improved by an optional deconvolution in x-space MPI but a determination of a sufficiently good convolution kernel is limited to 1D so far. Since the Chebyshev and x-space approach emanate from different domains as well as different reconstruction concepts, a link between the approaches is not obviously given. In this contribution we derive the mathematical formulas of both reconstruction techniques with same prerequisites, i.e. the field free point is moved on a sinusoidal trajectory. Regarding the performance, it can be shown that the x-space approach requires $O(N)$ arithmetic operations for the native image reconstruction compared to $O(N \log N)$ if an additional image deconvolution is applied. The number of operations for the Chebyshev reconstruction is $O(N \log N)$, i.e. it has the same computational effort as for x-space with deconvolution. Finally, we will show that, mathematically, x-space and Chebyshev reconstruction are identical and differ in the interpolation of data, only. The findings of the comparative study are a fundamental basis for the future development of 2D/3D models in MPI.

Corresponding Author: M. Ahlborg, ahlborg@imt.uni-Lübeck.de

References

[1] M. Gruettner, et al., "On the Formulation of the Image Reconstruction Problem in Magnetic Particle Imaging," Biomed Tech, vol. 58, no. 6, pp. 583 - 91, 2013.

[2] B. Gleich and J. Weizenecker, "Tomographic imaging using the nonlinear response of magnetic particles," Nature, vol. 435, no. 7046, pp.1214 - 1217, June 2005.

[3] T. Knopp, et al., "Model-based reconstruction for magnetic particle imaging," IEEE Trans. Med. Imaging, vol. 29, no. 1, pp. 12 - 18, 2010.

[4] J. Rahmer, et al., "Signal encoding in magnetic particle imaging," BMC Med. Imaging, vol. 9, 2009.

[5] P. Goodwill and S. Conolly, "Multi-dimensional x-space magnetic particle imaging," IEEE Trans. Med. Imag., vol. 30, no. 9, pp. 1581 - 1590, 2011.

Acknowledgements

We acknowledge the Federal Ministry of Education and Research, Germany under grant number 13N11090 as well as the European Union and the State Schleswig-Holstein (Program for the Future-Economy: 122-10-004).

Corresponding Author: M. Ahlborg, ahlborg@imt.uni-Lübeck.de

P21 SIMULATION STUDY ON ITERATIVE RECONSTRUCTION METHOD FOR TIME-CORRELATION MAGNETIC PARTICLE IMAGING WITH CONTINUOUS TRAJECTORY SCAN

Shota Shimizu[1], Takumi Homma[1], Hiroki Tsuchiya[2], Yasutoshi Ishihara[2]

[1]*Graduate School of Science and Technology, Meiji University, Kanagawa, Japan*
[2]*School of Science and Technology, Meiji University, Kanagawa, Japan*

In magnetic particle imaging (MPI), image artifacts and blurring in reconstructed images are caused by imperfections in the MPI system and certain properties of magnetic nanoparticles (MNPs) [1]. In order to overcome these problems, we have previously proposed a reconstruction method that utilizes the correlation information between the waveforms of the electromotive force generated from an MNP existing at a field-free point (FFP) and the electromotive force existing beyond the FFP [2]. By the use of this method, image artifacts were significantly reduced, and image reconstruction could be performed without the inverse-matrix operation used in conventional image reconstruction methods. However, this reconstruction method has two problems. The first is the problem of the lengthy scan time over the field of view (FOV), because every FFP is discretely scanned at each image matrix point. The second problem is image blurring in the reconstructed image that cannot be avoided in principle in this method. In order to solve these problems, in addition to the application of the continuous trajectory (Lissajous trajectory) scan method [3], we propose a new reconstruction method to improve the abovementioned correlation-based reconstruction method. The new reconstruction method is based on iteratively correcting image artifacts and blurring by reducing the difference between the observed signals from MNPs and the calculated waveforms for the reconstructed image. In particular, the waveforms of the electromotive force are firstly calculated at each matrix point (FFP) from an initially reconstructed image. Secondly, the difference (error) between the observed signals from MNPs at each FFP and the abovementioned calculated waveforms is determined. Finally, the corrected image components are estimated from this error, and subsequently, the image artifacts and blurring are corrected. These operations are iteratively performed. To confirm the effectiveness of this proposed method, numerical simulations were performed. In the simulations, two coil pairs were used to scan the FFP. The FOV was set to 10 [mm] × 10 [mm] with a matrix size of 35 × 35. A gradient magnetic field of 2.5 [T/m] was applied to MNPs with a particle diameter of 35 [nm]. In the simulation results (Fig. 1), although image blurring occurred upon using the correlation-based reconstruction method with the continuous trajectory scan, it was partly corrected by our proposed method. Moreover, the reconstruction results obtained via various methods (conventional (Fig. 1 (b)), our previous (Fig. 1 (c)), and proposed methods (Fig. 1 (d)) were compared under the abovementioned simulation conditions. We confirmed that the proposed method was more effective in suppressing image artifacts and blurring than the other methods. Futhermore, we confirmed that the proposed method exhibited higher tolerance with respect to noise than the other methods. However, since the results of the proposed method did not show satisfactory convergence during the iteration, image blurring still appeared in the reconstructed image. Therefore, the proposed method needs to be improved further in terms of reducing the convergence time and enhancing the image resolution.

Corresponding Author: S. Shimizu, ce32025@meiji.ac.jp

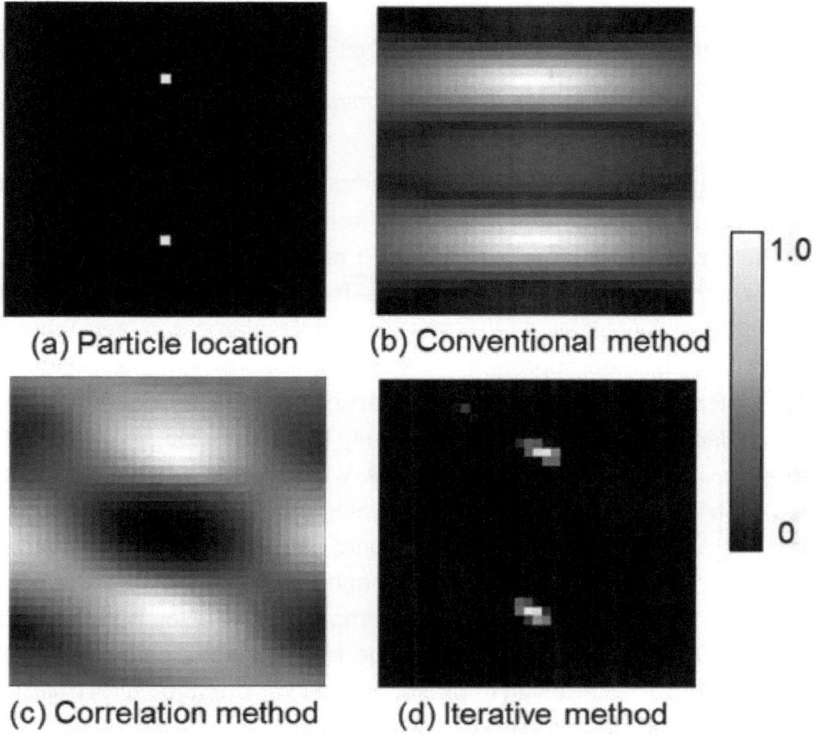

Figure 1 Reconstruction results by each method.

[1] B. Gleich, J. Weizenecker, "Tomographic imaging using the nonlinear response of magnetic particles." Nature, vol. 435, pp. 1214-1217, 2005.

[2] Y. Ishihara, T. Kuwabara, T. Honma, Y. Nakagawa "Correlation based image reconstruction methods for magnetic particle imaging." IEICE Trans. Inf. & Syst. E95-D (3), pp. 872-879, 2012.

[3] J. Weizenecker, J. Borgert and B. Gleich "A simulation study on the resolution and sensitivity of magnetic particle imaging." Phys. Med. Biol. 52(21), pp.6363-6374, 2007.

Corresponding Author: S. Shimizu, ce32025@meiji.ac.jp

P22 TRAJECTORY ANALYSIS USING PATCHES FOR MAGNETIC PARTICLE IMAGING

Patryk Szwargulski, Mandy Ahlborg, Christian Kaethner, Thorsten M. Buzug

Institute of Medical Engineering, University of Lübeck, Germany

Magnetic Particle Imaging (MPI) is an imaging technique based on the determination of magnetic material by moving a field free point along specified trajectories, which are used to sample the field of view (FOV) [1]. The coverage of large areas in MPI requires magnetic fields with high amplitudes. Thus, challenging research areas are the handling of safety limits, such as stimulation of the peripheral nervous system, or technical difficulties, as for example handling large data sets when performing image reconstruction. A recently published approach to address the aforementioned issues is to separate the FOV into small FOV patches, each covering just a part of the FOV to reduce the field amplitudes [2]. Such patches are sampled and reconstructed separately and combined afterwards. To reduce artifacts it is possible to use an overlap of the individual patches, which has to be post processed [2, 3]. Although different trajectories for MPI were investigated concerning image quality, so far, trajectory studies with FOV patches are based on the Lissajous trajectory, only. The aim of this work is to analyze the effect of different trajectories combined with the patch approach. In this study, the FOV is separated into four patches, which are separately reconstructed. The sampling time of all patches is chosen to be the same as for the whole FOV, i.e. the coverage with one large trajectory. In a simulation study, multiple trajectories, i.e. the cartesian, the cartesian improved, the radial, and the spiral trajectory, are compared with the Lissajous trajectory [4]. In addition, a new patch formation of the radial trajectory based on a phase shift between each of the patches is introduced (see Figure 1). As a result of the phase shift, the spikes of the radial trajectories interlock, to use the given space in an optimal way. As a follow-up, an empiric study is performed to analyze the influence of overlapped patches on each trajectory combined with two different post-processing methods. An overlap of the patches is a preventive measure to prohibit arising truncation artifacts. As a result, an optimal overlap for each trajectory is found and it is shown that for all trajectories an artifact correction is possible using overlapped patches. It can be shown that the Lissajous trajectory, which is mostly used for MPI, provides satisfactory results. However, the results of overlapped patches with a circular shaped trajectory increase the spatial resolution (see Figure 1). The results of the studies in this work are an important step to realize an optimal use of trajectory patches for MPI.

Corresponding Author: P. Szwargulski, szwargulski@imt.uni-Lübeck.de

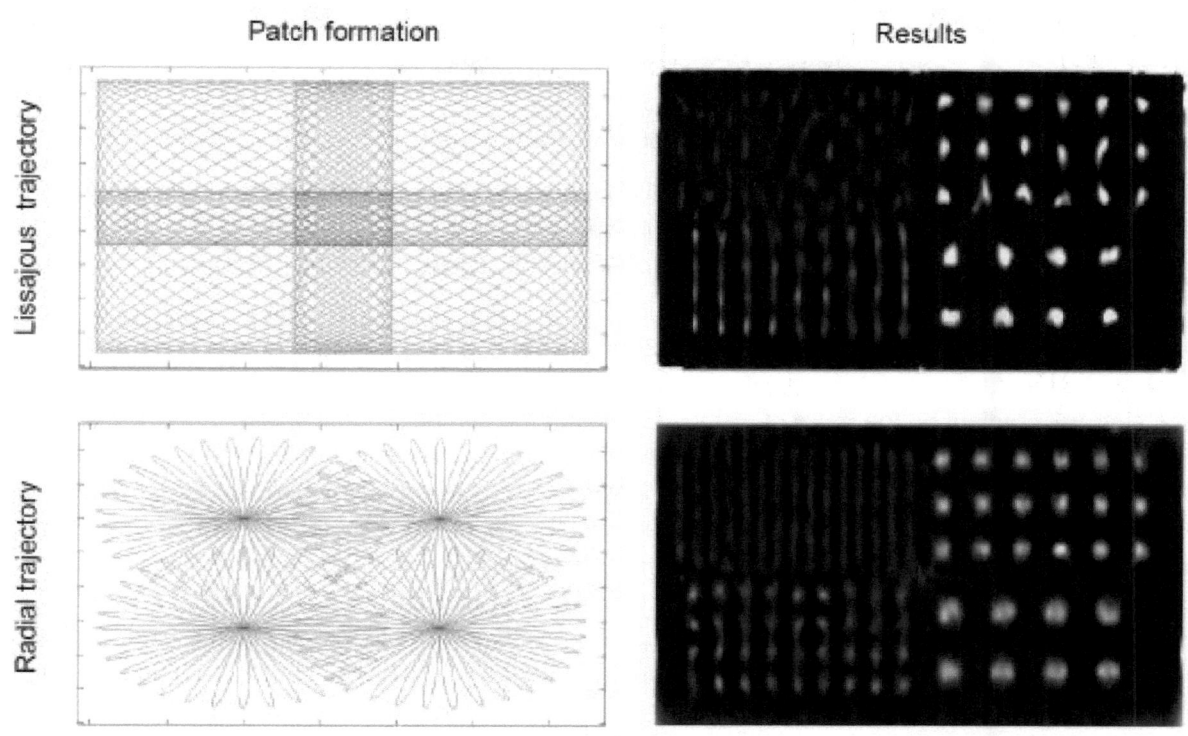

Figure 1: Results for the Lissajous and radial trajectory using a 10% overlap for the patches and a cut-off as post processing method. It is shown that applying the radial trajectory increases the spatial resolution compared to the Lissajous trajectory.

[1] B. Gleich and J. Weizenecker. Tomographic Imaging Using the Nonlinear Response of Magnetic Particles. Nature, 435(7046):1214-1217, 2005.

[2] M. Gruettner, T. F. Sattel, M. Graeser, H. Wojtczyk, G. Bringout, W. Tenner, and T. M. Buzug. Enlarging the Field of View in Magnetic Particle Imaging - A Comparison. Springer Proceedings in Physics, 140:249-253, 2012.

[3] J. Rahmer, B. Gleich, C. Bontus, I. Schmale, J. Schmidt, J. Kanzenbach, O. Woywode, J. Weizenecker, and J. Borgert. Results on Rapid 3D Magnetic Particle Imaging with a Large Field of View. Proceedings of the International Society for Magnetic Resonance in Medicine, 19:629, 2011.

[4] T. Knopp, S. Biederer, T. Sattel, J. Weizenecker, B. Gleich, J. Borgert, and T. M. Buzug. Trajectory Analysis for Magnetic Particle Imaging. Physics in Medicine and Biology, 54(2):385-97, 2009.

Corresponding Author: P. Szwargulski, szwargulski@imt.uni-Lübeck.de

P23 SIMULATING AND MODELING RELAXATION EFFECTS IN MAGNETIC PARTICLE IMAGING

Martin A. Rückert[1,3], Patrick Vogel[1,2,3], Peter M. Jakob[1,2], Volker C. Behr[1]

[1]Department of Experimental Physics 5 (Biophysics), University of Würzburg, Germany
[2]Research Center for Magnetic Resonance Bavaria e.V. (MRB), Würzburg, Germany
[3]Institute of Medical Engineering, University of Applied Sciences Würzburg-Schweinfurt, Germany

Magnetic Particle Imaging (MPI) was first published in 2005 [1]. It is based on the nonlinear response of ferro- and superparamagnetic materials to varying magnetic fields. For imaging a field free point (FFP) with a strong gradient on the order of is moved through the sample. Signal arises only in the vicinity of the FFP. Simulating this imaging process is currently based on the Langevin function [2], i.e. relaxation effects are completely ignored. MPI applies relatively high frequencies where relaxation effects are no longer negligible [3]. The theory and experimental data in [4] indicate that relaxation decreases the signal-to-noise ratio and blurs the image in the scanning direction. It is therefore important for an accurate MPI signal simulation to also account for relaxation effects.

The most general description for magnetic particle systems in time-varying fields is the Langevin equation which calculates the dynamic of the individual particle. The disadvantage of this approach is the huge numerical burden. For simulating suspensions of magnetic nanoparticles, at least averages are necessary for a statistical error below .

The presented work derives an approximation for directly calculating the average of the macroscopic magnetization. This is similar to the Fokker-Planck equation which is solved for alternating magnetic fields [5], but hard to solve for the general case. The presented approximation aims at the general description for arbitrary magnetic vector fields necessary for simulating MPI in 3D. The approximation yields accurate results for offset fields that are parallel to the alternating field (1D case – fig 1, middle).

The derivation for 3D fields yields promising results except for orthogonal offset fields smaller than of the alternating field, where it yields non-physical results. The approximation for 1D was about times faster in comparison to averages of the Langevin equation, for 3D it was about times faster (using Matlab, Mathworks Natick, MA, USA).

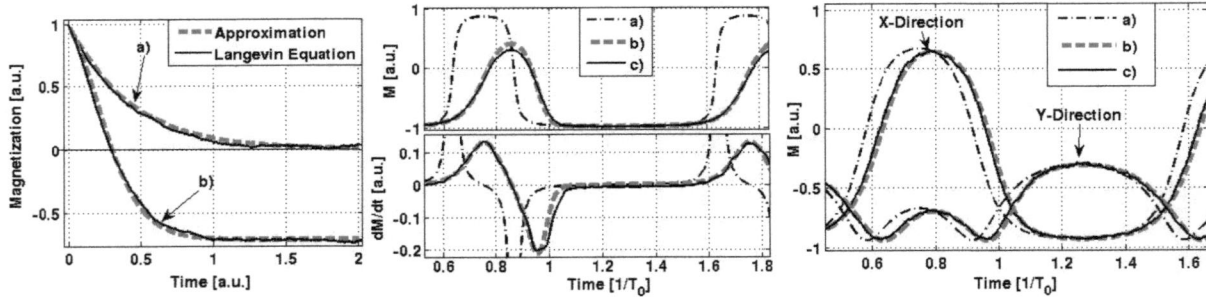

Fig. 1: Left: Simulating relaxation into equilibrium: results using the approximation and the Langevin equation (10^3 averages) for a) zero-field, b) with negative offsetfield. Middle: Magnetization and its time-derivative in an alternating field (periodic time) and an offsetfield, calculated with a) Langevin function, b) approximation, c) Langevin equation. Right: Simulating in offset fields with orthogonal components: a) Langevin function, b) Langevin equation, c) approximation. The excitation field oscillates in x-direction, the offset field is oriented diagonal in x- and y-direction.

Corresponding Author: M. Rückert, Martin.Rückert@physik.uni-Würzburg.de

[1] B. Gleich, and J. Weizenecker, "Tomographic imaging using the nonlinear response of magnetic particles", Nature 435, 1214-1217, Jun. 2005.

[2] Goodwill PW, Conolly SM. Multidimensional X-space magnetic particle imaging. IEEE Trans Med Imaging 2011; 30: 1581–1590.

[3] Goodwill PW, Tamrazian A, Croft LR, et al. Ferrohydrodynamic relaxometry for magnetic particle imaging. Appl Phys Lett 2011; 98: 262502.

[4] Croft LR, Goodwill PW, Conolly SM. Relaxation in x-space magnetic particle imaging. IEEE Trans Med Imaging 2012; 28: 2335–2342.

[5] Yoshida T, Enpuku K. Simulation and quantitative clarification of AC susceptibility of magnetic fluid in nonlinear Brownian relaxation region. Jpn J Appl Phys 2009; 48: 127002.

Corresponding Author: M. Rückert, Martin.Rückert@physik.uni-Würzburg.de

P24 EVALUATION OF QUANTITY AND LINEARITY WITH REGARD TO TIKHONOV REGULARIZATION, NUMBER OF ITERATIONS AND SELECTION OF FREQUENCY COMPONENTS IN THE MPI RECONSTRUCTION PROCESS

Alexander Weber[1], Jochen Franke[1], Jürgen Weizenecker[2], Ulrich Heinen[1], Michael Heidenreich[1], Wolfgang Ruhm[1], Thorsten M. Buzug[3]

[1]Bruker BioSpin MRI GmbH, Ettlingen, Germany
[2]University of Applied Siences, Karlsruhe, Germany
[3]Institute of Medical Engineering, University of Lübeck, Germany

Magnetic particle imaging (MPI) is a new imaging modality which allows the detection of superparamagnetic iron oxide nanoparticles in vivo in three dimensions and in real time. Furthermore, the physical theory predicts a quantitative measurement.

One approach to reconstruct the particle distribution is the system function method. In this method a linear system of equations has to be solved. Hereby the system matrix of the linear system describes the mapping between the MPI image and the signals induced in the receive coils.

Commonly the system matrix is determined by a calibration scan, where the system response of a small delta sample with the size of approximately one voxel is measured at the various discretization positions of the field-of-view (FOV).

As the system matrix exhibits a high condition number and both the system matrix and the measurement signal contain noise, the Tikhonov regularization is introduced to solve the linear system of equations.

Thereby a regularization parameter λ is introduced, which weights the solution in comparison to the residual. Decreasing λ improves the spatial resolution of the reconstructed particle map, however it increases also the signal-to-noise ratio and thus the best trade-off between resolution and noise has to be found.

Furthermore, the linear system of equations is huge and thus iterative algorithms are necessary to solve this problem. Hereby the Kaczmarz algorithm shows good performance for the MPI reconstruction problem. Again, the number of iterations influences the reconstruction result. Increasing the number of iterations beyond a certain degree leads to overfitting of the solution to noise, but computing insufficient iterations does not provide the best possible reconstruction result.

In addition, the selection of the trustful frequency components has also an effect to the reconstruction of the particle distribution.

In this work, the effect of the number of iterations, the regularization parameter and the selection of the frequency components on the reconstruction result is investigated with regard to the quantity and the linearity of the signal intensities.

Corresponding Author: A. Weber, Alexander.Weber@bruker-biospin.de

P25 MAGNETIC PARTICLES IMAGE RECONSTRUCT THROUGH JACOBI SINGULAR VALUE DECOMPOSITION

Su Rijian[1], Guo Gongbing[1], Zhang Qiuwen[1], Gan Yong[1], Huang Zhen[2] Zhong Jing[2], Du Zhongzhou[2]

[1]School of Computer&Communication engineering, Zhengzhou University of Light Industry, China
[2]School of Automation, Huazhong University of Science and Technology, Wuhan, China

Magnetic Particle Imaging is a novel imaging modality which makes use of the nonlinear magnetization characteristics of the superparamagnetic iron-oxide nanoparticles(SPIOs)[1]. To reconstruct the image, the spatial or temporal distribution of SPIOs must to be quantitatively measured. According to the Langevintheory, the main reconstruction step is to solve the concentration of SPIOs, i.e. to solve the linear system of equations between the received Fourier transformed voltage signal and concentrationof SPIOs. Aiming for imaging with high spatial resolutionand a large field of view, the number of equations grows rapidly and especially the handling of the system function becomes challenging. This paper proposes a Jacobi algorithm for the singular value decomposition (SVD) of system function matrix. Different from traditional SVD approach, the improved algorithm eventually transfers the system function matrix to product of orthogonal matrix and diagonal matrix through a series of Jacobi rotations. In addition, Jacobi algorithm has adequate resolution and fast speed. Simulation results show that the algorithm has very good performance in magnetic particle image reconstruction.

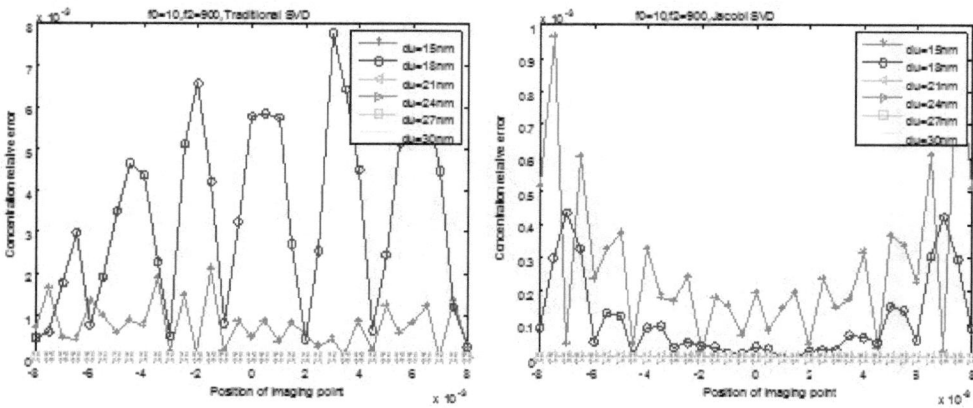

[1] Buzug TM, Bringout G, Erbe M, Gräfe K, Graeser M, Gruettner M, Halkola A, Sattel TF, Tenner W, Wojtczyk H, Haegele J, Vogt FM, Barkhausen J, Lüdtke-Buzug K. Magnetic particle imaging: introduction to imaging and hardware realization. Z Med Phys. 2012 Dec;22(4):323-34.

[2] Gleich B, Weizenecker J. Tomographic imaging using the nonlinear response of magnetic particles. Nature. 2005 Jun 30;435(7046):1214-7.

[3] Drmac Z. A Posteriori Computation of the Singular Vectors in a Preconditioned Jacobi SVD Algorithm. IMA J. Numer. Anal. 1999, 19(2):191–213.

[4] Rahmer J, Weizenecker J, Gleich B, Borgert J. Signal encoding in magnetic particle imaging: properties of the system function. BMC Med Imaging. 2009 Apr 1;9:4.

Corresponding Author: S.Rijian,zzsrj@126.com

P26 — A FLEXIBLE AND MODULAR MPI SIMULATION FRAMEWORK AND ITS USE IN MODELLING A μMPI

Marcel Straub[1], Fabian Kiessling[2], Volkmar Schulz[1,3]

[1]*Physics of Molecular Imaging Systems (ExMI), Medical Faculty RWTH-Aachen University, Germany*
[2]*Experimental Molecular Imaging (ExMI), Medical Faculty RWTH-Aachen University, Germany*
[3]*Philips Research Europe, Aachen, Germany*

The availability of thorough system simulations for detailed and accurate performance prediction and optimization of existing and future designs for a new modality such as MPI (cf. [1]) are very important. Since there exists no freely available simulation framework for MPI yet, we are developing a modular and extensible framework. Our framework aims to simulate a complete MPI system by providing a description of all (drive and receive) coils, permanent magnet configurations, magnetic nanoparticle (MNP) distributions, and characteristics of the signal processing chain. In a first realization, the simulation is performed on a user defined spatial and temporal discrete grid. Currently, the magnetization of the MNP is modelled by either the Langevin (cf. [2]) theory or as ideal particles with infinite steepness at B=0 mT and ideal saturation. The magnetic fields are approximated in first order by calculating the Biot-Savart integral. Additionally the coupling constants between the excitation coils (e.g. drive field coils) and the receive coils can be determined. All coils can be described by an XML description language based on primitive geometric shapes or by using an externally created CAD description. Permanent magnets are implemented by using the "Equivalent Sources Method" (cf. [3]).

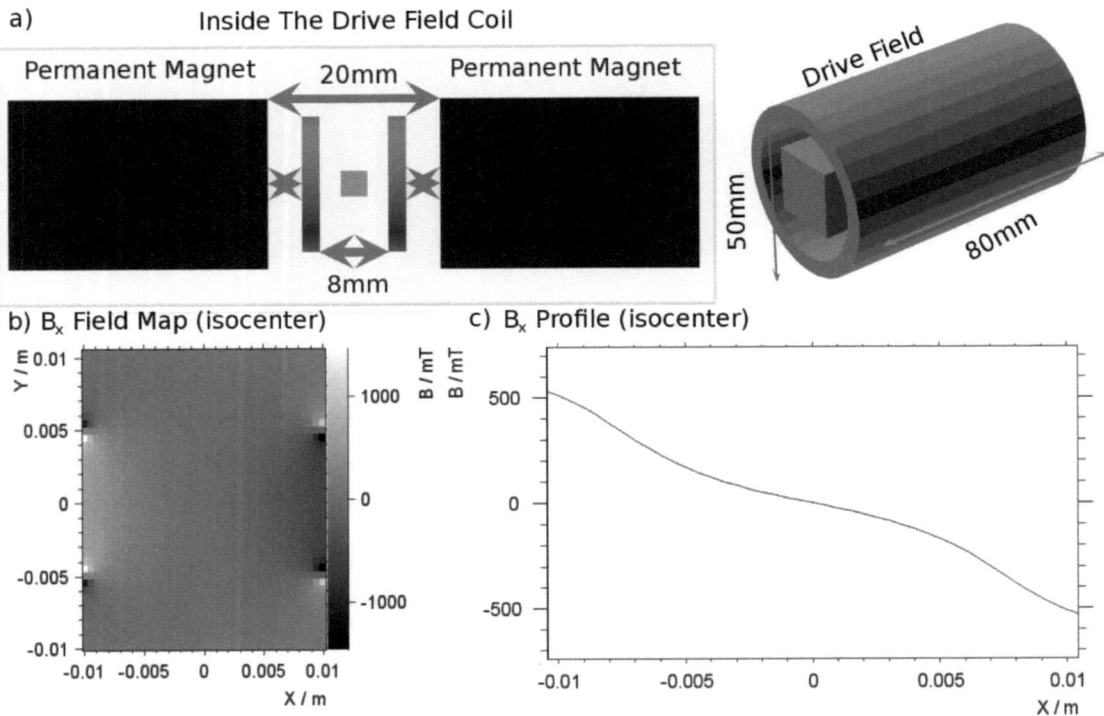

Fig. 1 a) Schematic of the μMPI scanner. The drive field encloses the probe and receive coils as well as the gradient field generator. b+c) Simulated gradient field map of B_x in the central plane.

Corresponding Author: M. Straub, marcel.straub@pmi.rwth-aachen.de

First simulations of a modelled µMPI system are shown. Thereby µMPI refers to a small one-dimensional system for samples of a size of a few tens of a cubic millimeter. A schematic view of the scanner is shown in Fig. 1a. For a scanner of this size permanent magnets are sufficient for creating a steep gradient field of 50 – 100 Tm^{-1} μ_0^{-1} (cf. [4]) which theoretically allows for a targeted spatial resolution of about (cf. [5]). First simulations show (cf. Fig. 1b,c) that with two permanent magnets (each 10×10×10 mm^3) with a magnetic field of 540 mT at the surface a gradient of about 54 Tm^{-1} μ_0^{-1} can be achieved. Even higher gradient strengths can be achieved by using permanent magnets of a different shape (e.g. "thicker" in the direction of the magnetization). The drive field is designed to scan a field of view of about 3 x 3 x 3 mm^3.

Acknowledgement:

The authors would like to thank Philips for their financial support of the Ph.D. position of Marcel Straub and for the useful discussions with Bernhard Gleich.

[1] B. Gleich and J. Weizenecker, "Tomographic imaging using the nonlinear response of magnetic particles.," *Nature*, vol. 435, no. 7046, pp. 1214–1217, Jun. 2005.

[2] S. Biederer, T. Knopp, T. F. Sattel, K. Lüdtke-Buzug, B. Gleich, J. Weizenecker, J. Borgert, and T. M. Buzug, "Magnetization response spectroscopy of superparamagnetic nanoparticles for magnetic particle imaging," *J. Phys. D. Appl. Phys.*, vol. 42, no. 20, p. 205007, Oct. 2009.

[3] S. Bobbio, F. Delfino, P. Girdinio, and P. Molfino, "Equivalent sources methods for the numerical evaluation of magnetic force with extension to nonlinear materials," *IEEE Trans. Magn.*, vol. 36, no. 4, pp. 663–666, Jul. 2000.

[4] J. M. D. Coey, "Permanent magnet applications," *J. Magn. Magn. Mater.*, vol. 248, no. 3, pp. 441–456, Aug. 2002.

[5] P. W. Goodwill, E. U. Saritas, L. R. Croft, T. N. Kim, K. M. Krishnan, D. V. Schaffer, and S. M. Conolly, "X-Space MPI: Magnetic Nanoparticles for Safe Medical Imaging," *Adv. Mater.*, vol. 24, no. 28, pp. 3870–3877, Jul. 2012.

Corresponding Author: M. Straub, marcel.straub@pmi.rwth-aachen.de

P27 MAGNETIC FIELD SIMULATION TOOLBOX FOR MPI MODELING

Waldemar T. Smolik, Przemysław R. Wróblewski, Jan Szyszko

Institute of Radioelectronics, Warsaw University of Technology, Poland

In this paper we present the progress in the development of the software for numerical modeling of magnetic particle imaging. The modeling software will enable to evaluate new concepts in the design of MPI scanner. Our group is developing a MPI scanner setup for small animals or samples. We already build test setup with coils for two dimensional imaging (Fig. 1b). The modeling of magnetic field distribution can facilitate the design of the coil setup for a scanner. Though there are available many commercial and open source programs for electromagnetic field modeling we are developing a custom solver dedicated to MPI in MATLAB environment. The numerical three dimensional solver is based on the finite volume method (FVM) and uses structural regular mesh for space discretization. Instead of differential formulation FVM involves a discretization of the integral formulation of the conservation laws in the physical space and offers advantages in algorithm implementation e.g. for local grid refinement. In the first version of our toolbox the state equation was solved using the iterative method. Additionally the homogeneous distribution of magnetic permeability was assumed for simplification of calculations. The new version of solver is based on Krylov space methods and sparse matrices. It enables three dimensional modeling of non-uniform permeability distribution. The advantage of Krylov space methods is that they enable relatively faster computation using sparse matrices compared to specialized Gauss elimination solvers for band diagonal matrices. Different Krylov methods, such as Conjugate Gradient method (CG), Biconjugate Gradient method (BiCG), Conjugate Gradient Squared method (CGS), Induced Dimension Reduction method (IDRS) were considered and tested.

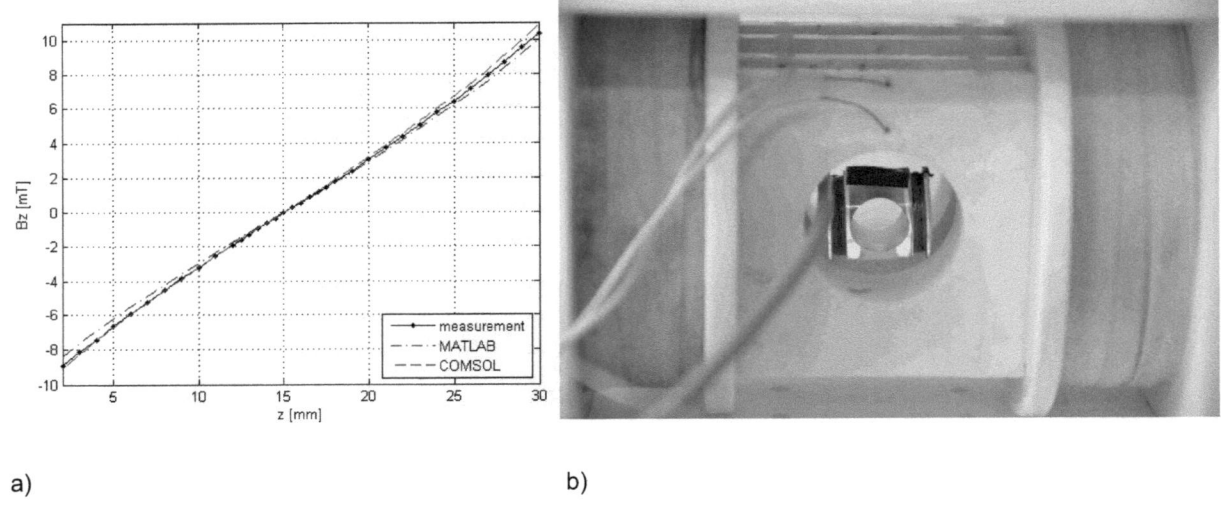

a) b)

Fig. 1 a) Magnetic gradient field distribution along Z axis (Bz component). Exemplary results of magnetic field simulation and measurement; b) Setup of two pairs of coils. Large coils shown on both sides are selection and driving coils for Z axis, while between them selection coils for Y axis are located. Receiving coil is visible inside a FOV of the scanner model.

The magnetic field simulations would be compared with COMSOL FEM software and measurements of magnetic field performed using the coil setup designed for a small MPI scanner (Fig. 1a). This setup consists of two pairs of Helmholtz coils for gradient and excitation field generation. Selection coils were able to generate gradient field with strength of about 0.4 T/m while fed with current of about 2.5 A. Using this setup already some experiments were conducted.

Corresponding Author: W. Smolik, W.Smolik@ire.pw.edu.pl

Detection of superparamagnetic particles was performed using 2nd and 3rd harmonics analyzes, as well as manual measurements of distribution of concentration of particles along one axis. New solver is being developed to better simulate magnetic field distribution of our experimental coils setup and measurements performed with it. Our new implementation would allow faster calculations and more accurate results.

References

[1] GUTKNECHT, Martin H. A brief introduction to Krylov space methods for solving linear systems. In: *Frontiers of Computational Science*. Springer Berlin Heidelberg, 2007. p. 53-62.

[2] SONNEVELD, Peter; VAN GIJZEN, Martin B. IDR (s): A family of simple and fast algorithms for solving large nonsymmetric systems of linear equations. *SIAM Journal on Scientific Computing*, 2008, 31.2: 1035-1062.

[3] VAN DER VORST, Henk A. Bi-CGSTAB: A fast and smoothly converging variant of Bi-CG for the solution of nonsymmetric linear systems. *SIAM Journal on scientific and Statistical Computing*, 1992, 13.2: 631-644.

[4] SMOLIK, Waldemar T.; WROBLEWSKI, Przemyslaw R.; SZYSZKO, Jan. Numerical modeling of magnetic field for magnetic particle imaging. In: *Imaging Systems and Techniques (IST), 2012 IEEE International Conference on*. IEEE, 2012. p. 436-441.

Corresponding Author: W. Smolik, W.Smolik@ire.pw.edu.pl

Poster

MPI Theory, Relaxometry, Magnetometry

P28 ROTATIONAL DRIFT SPECTROSCOPY FOR MAGNETIC PARTICLE ENSEMBLES

Martin A. Rückert[1,3], Patrick Vogel[1,2,3], Anna Vilter[1,2], Walter H. Kullmann[3], Peter M. Jakob[1,2], Volker C. Behr[1]

[1]*Department of Experimental Physics 5 (Biophysics), University of Würzburg, Germany*
[2]*Research Center for Magnetic Resonance Bavaria e.V. (MRB), Würzburg, Germany*
[3]*Institute of Medical Engineering, University of Applied Sciences Würzburg-Schweinfurt, Germany*

A new method for characterizing magnetic particle ensembles and first measurements are presented. Rotational drift spectroscopy (RDS) is based on the asynchronous rotational drift of magnetic particles in rotating magnetic fields. The rotational drift has been measured on single particles [1]. In respect of large ensembles of magnetic particles, the steady state susceptibility in rotating field has been studied [2]. The presented method aims at measuring rotational drift behavior on magnetic particle ensembles in rotating fields. In order to do so, the system needs to be driven out of its steady-state distribution, e.g. by applying a short unipolar magnetic pulse. This aligns the magnetic moments of all particles and results in a transient rotating macroscopic magnetization. It decays due to disturbances like rotational diffusion, very similar to the magnetization decay in magnetorelaxometry [3]. It also decays due to differences in rotational drift rates for different particles. The later effect can be reversed by changing the rotating direction of the rotating field.

In the experiment two orthogonal coil pairs (fig. 1 left) where driven with two different frequencies f_1=57.6 kHz and f_2=50.2 kHz.. The resulting rotating magnetic field periodically changes its rotating direction with a frequency of $(f_1-f_2)/2$=3.7 kHz, resulting in a train of signal echoes with the same frequency. The rotating field started ~3 ms after a magnetic pulse. The induction of the rotating field was separated from the signal by using a 5th-order Chebychev low-pass filter. The initial magnetic pulse would cause oscillations in the low-pass that are much higher than the typical signal. It was suppressed from the receiver chain by using an electro-mechanical switch.

Measurements were performed on different materials. Shown in fig. 1 are: a) iron swarfs in water (size: ~100 µm), b) silica particles with maghemite, diameter: ~500 nm (SiMAG-Silanol, chemicell, Berlin, Germany), c) plain iron oxid nanoparticles, diameter: ~200 nm (iron oxide 200 nm, micromod, Rostock, Germany), e) dextran coated magnetite particles, diameter: ~250 nm (PMC-250, Kisker, Steinfurt, Germany). All shown particles were highly aggregated and show different signals caused by their structure, hysteresis, shape, core-size, etc.

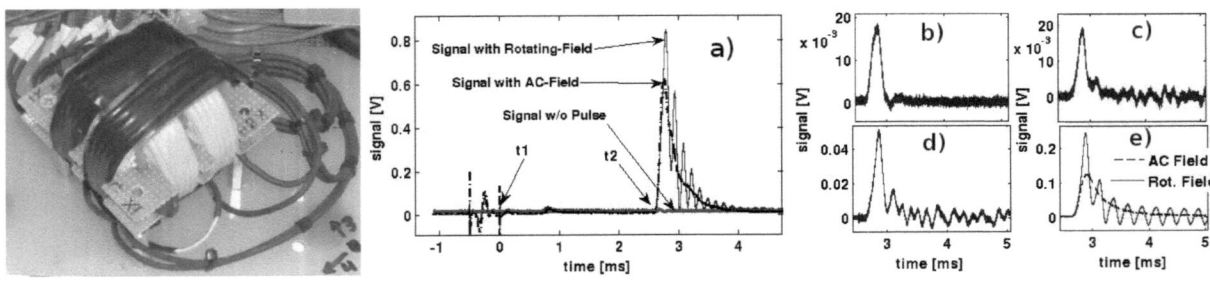

Fig. 1: Left: Coil system for generating the rotating field. Pulse- and receiver coil are inside. Sample diameter: 5mm. Right: a) Pulse suppression ends at t1 (Pulse starts 500µs before t1, FHWM: 20µs, Peak value: 200mT). Rotating field starts at t2. Strength of rotating field: a) 750µT, b) – e) 15mT. Dash-dotted line in a) and dashed line e): only a linearly alternating magnetic field was applied.

Corresponding Author: M. Rückert, Martin.Rückert@physik.uni-Würzburg.de

[1] B. McNaughton et al., "Physiochemical microparticle sensors based on nonlinear magnetic oscillations", Sensors and Actuators B 121 330–340 (2007).

[2] J. Dieckhoff, M. Schilling, and F. Ludwig, „Fluxgate based detection of magnetic nanoparticle dynamics in a rotating magnetic field", Appl. Phys. Letters 99, 112501-1 – 3 (2011).

[3] E Heim et al., "Binding assays with streptavidin-functionalized superparamagnetic nanoparticles and biotinylated analytes using fluxgate magnetorelaxometry", J. Magn. Magn. Mater 321, 1628–1631 (2009).

Corresponding Author: M. Rückert, Martin.Rückert@physik.uni-Würzburg.de

P29 SIMULATING THE SIGNAL GENERATION OF ROTATIONAL DRIFT SPECTROSCOPY

Martin A. Rückert[1,3], Patrick Vogel[1,2,3], Thomas Kampf[1], Walter H. Kullmann[3], Peter M. Jakob[1,2], Volker C. Behr[1]

[1]*Department of Experimental Physics 5 (Biophysics), University of Würzburg, Germany*
[2]*Research Center for Magnetic Resonance Bavaria e.V. (MRB), Würzburg, Germany*
[3]*Institute of Medical Engineering, University of Applied Sciences Würzburg-Schweinfurt, Germany*

A new method for characterizing magnetic particle ensembles and first measurements are presented. Rotational drift spectroscopy (RDS) is based on the asynchronous rotational drift of magnetic particles in rotating magnetic fields. The rotational drift has been measured on single particles [1]. In respect of large ensembles of magnetic particles, the steady state susceptibility in rotating field has been studied [2]. The presented method aims at measuring rotational drift behavior on magnetic particle ensembles in rotating fields. In order to do so, the system needs to be driven out of its steady-state distribution, e.g. by applying a short unipolar magnetic pulse. This aligns the magnetic moments of all particles and results in a transient rotating macroscopic magnetization. It decays due to disturbances like rotational diffusion, very similar to the magnetization decay in magnetorelaxometry [3]. It also decays due to differences in rotational drift rates for different particles which can be reversed by changing the rotating direction of the rotating field.

The presented simulation study and analysis aims at evaluating the possibilities of RDS. The study is currently limited to systems consisting of non-interacting spherical magnetic particles. Fig. 1 (a) illustrates the strong field dependency of the rotational drift frequency. Fig. 1 (b) and (c) shows the generation of a signal echo. Preliminary experiments that demonstrate signal echoes have been performed (measuring the envelope of the signal echo without being able to resolve the rotational drift frequency directly). The behavior of such systems is very promising for enabling bio-sensing applications similar to magnetorelaxometry [3], yet possibly with higher sensitivity, a much shorter measurement time scale and the possibility of accessing additional particle properties like particle shape, inter-particle coupling and the ratio between magnetic moment and rotational friction.

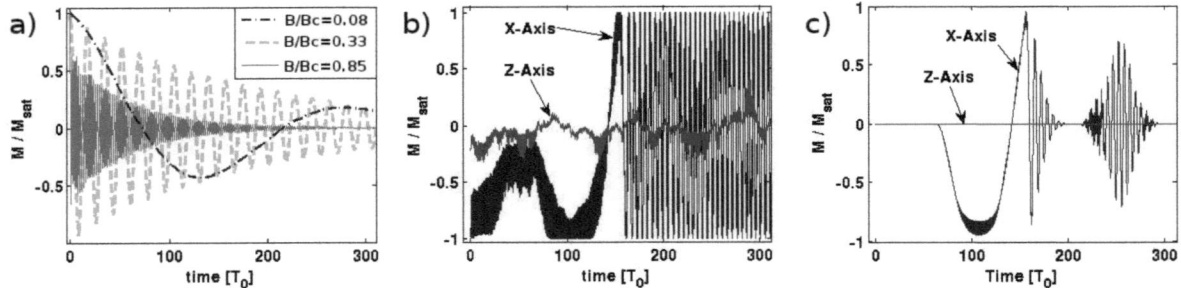

Fig. 1 (a): Rotational drift magnetization decay for different rotating magnetic field strengths B. Bc refers to the critical field strengths. The time is given in terms of the periodic time T_0 of the rotating field. (b): Simulating the magnetization of a single particle in an exemplary rotating magnetic field sequence suitable for RDS. Shown is the magnetization in x- (blue), y- (green) and z- direction. The rotating plane is the x- and y-plane. The initial pulse is applied between $\tau = 80T_0 ... 120T_0$. (c): Simulation of a particle system with 10^5 non-interacting magnetic particles with Gaussian distributed $B/Bc=0.5 \pm 0.05$. The rotating direction is inverted at $t= 200\ T_0$ which shows no effect in (b), but yields a signal echo in (c). Frequency components of the external field are filtered in (c).

Corresponding Author: M. Rückert, Martin.Rückert@physik.uni-Würzburg.de

[1] B. McNaughton et al., "Physiochemical microparticle sensors based on nonlinear magnetic oscillations", Sensors and Actuators B 121 330–340 (2007).

[2] J. Dieckhoff, M. Schilling, and F. Ludwig, „Fluxgate based detection of magnetic nanoparticle dynamics in a rotating magnetic field", Appl. Phys. Letters 99, 112501-1 – 3 (2011).

[3] E Heim et al., "Binding assays with streptavidin-functionalized superparamagnetic nanoparticles and biotinylated analytes using fluxgate magnetorelaxometry", J. Magn. Magn. Mater 321, 1628–1631 (2009).

Corresponding Author: M. Rückert, Martin.Rückert@physik.uni-Würzburg.de

P30 MAGNETIC PARTICLE SPECTROSCOPY TO DETERMINE THE MAGNETIC DRUG TARGETING EFFICIENCY OF DIFFERENT MAGNETIC NANOPARTICLES IN A FLOW PHANTOM

Patricia Radon[1], Maik Liebl[1], Nadine Pömpner[2], Marcus Stapf[2], Frank Wiekhorst[1], Kurt Gitter[3], Ingrid Hilger[2], Stefan Odenbach[3], Lutz Trahms[1]

[1]*Physikalisch-Technische Bundesanstalt, Berlin, Germany*
[2]*Institute of Diagnostic and Interventional Radiology I, Universitätsklinikum Jena, Germany*
[3]*Institut fuer Strömungsmechanik, Technische Universität Dresden, Germany*

Biomedical applications of magnetic nanoparticles (MNP) as contrast agents, drug carriers or heat production in the blood flow of organisms or humans are presently intensively investigated. To select suitable MNP for a preclinical combined magnetic drug targeting/hyperthermia study in a tumor mouse model we built up a simple flow phantom. Magnetic Particle Spectroscopy (MPS) serves as a sensitive detection technique to quantify the accumulated MNP amount in a sample after magnetic targeting (MT). In pilot experiments we demonstrate the performance of our setup to quantify the retention of MNP by magnetic targeting under controlled physiological blood flow and MNP concentration conditions.

The MT flow phantom consisted of a peristaltic pump with fixed inlet and outlet tubes, a small cubic neodymium magnet, a reservoir for MNP suspension input and a removable retention tube of 1 mm inner diameter. We used hydroxyethyl starch coated MNP of 50 nm, 200 nm and 300 nm mean hydrodynamic diameter (chemicell, Berlin) diluted in 0.1% bovine serum albumin to an clinically tolerable iron concentration (7.5 mmol/l). In addition, we performed MT also in EDTA stabilized human blood using the 200 nm MNP. The suspension was pumped with a flow rate of 350 µl/ min through the flow system and the targeting magnet had a fixed distance to the retention tube. After defined time intervals (t_{MT} = 1, 5, 10, 30, 100, 1000 min), 10 µl aliquots from the retention tube and the reservoir were taken to determine the iron concentration by means of MPS. MPS employs the nonlinear magnetic response of MNP exposed to a strong oscillating magnetic field (up to 25 mT at 25 kHz), while biological tissue and paramagnetic blood iron do not contribute.

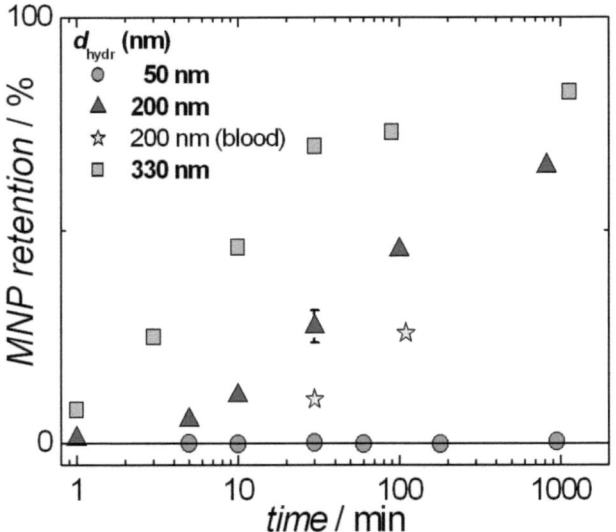

Fig 1: MNP retention as a function of MT-time for MNP of three different hydrodynamic diameters. The input concentration (7.5 mmol/l) was the same for all MNP.

Corresponding Author: P. Radon, patricia.radon@ptb.de

As expected the MT yield is crucially determined by the hydrodynamic diameter d_{hydr} (Fig 1). For d_{hydr} = 50 nm MNP we found nearly no retention (<1% even after 1000 min), while for d_{hydr} = 330 nm MNP after 30 min about 70% of the MNP were accumulated and the retention process showed already a saturation behavior for longer times t_{MT}. For d_{hydr} = 200 nm the retention is only about 25% at 30 min and reaches about 65% at 1000 min. For d_{hydr} = 200 nm in blood, the retention is further reduced to about 10%, probably due to the higher viscosity. Changes in the shape of the MPS spectrum indicate a moderate increase of larger MNP in the retention tube during MT. These alterations in the size distribution were confirmed by magnetorelaxometry measurements of the same samples.

We demonstrate with our setup the quantitative assessment of magnetic targeting efficiency of MNP at biologically tolerable (clinical) concentrations. Using different tube diameters or flow rates and tube materials together with variations of the flow rate and magnetic field gradients this allows for controlled investigations of physical and physiological properties during MT. In a next step we will incorporate a dedicated targeting magnet with defined gradients developed for mice tumor studies.

Corresponding Author: P. Radon, patricia.radon@ptb.de

P31 — FRAMEWORK TO CHARACTERIZE MPI TRACERS IN TERMS OF ACHIEVABLE RESOLUTION, FOV AND SPECTRAL DETECTION LIMIT

Florian Palmetshofer, Daniel Schmidt, Uwe Steinhoff

Physikalisch-Technische Bundesanstalt, Berlin, Germany

The goal of this work is to develop a framework for characterizing MPI tracer material with respect to detection limit, spatial resolution and field of view (FOV) at given drive field amplitudes. The detection limit of an MPI tracer material in an MPI scanner is the minimum magnetic nanoparticle (MNP) amount generating a signal above the harmonic noise level. It is important to know the detection limit separately for each higher harmonic, since the number of harmonics relates to the spatial resolution in image reconstruction.

If the iron amount per voxel is higher than the detection limit for a specific harmonic, this harmonic can be detected from that voxel. The voxel length Δx in one direction of the reconstructed tracer distribution depends on the field of view $2H/G$ and on the maximum number k of investigated harmonics by approximately $\Delta x \sim H/G \cdot 1/k$. Here H is the drive field amplitude and G is the gradient strength. This dependence is shown for the third harmonic in Fig. 1.

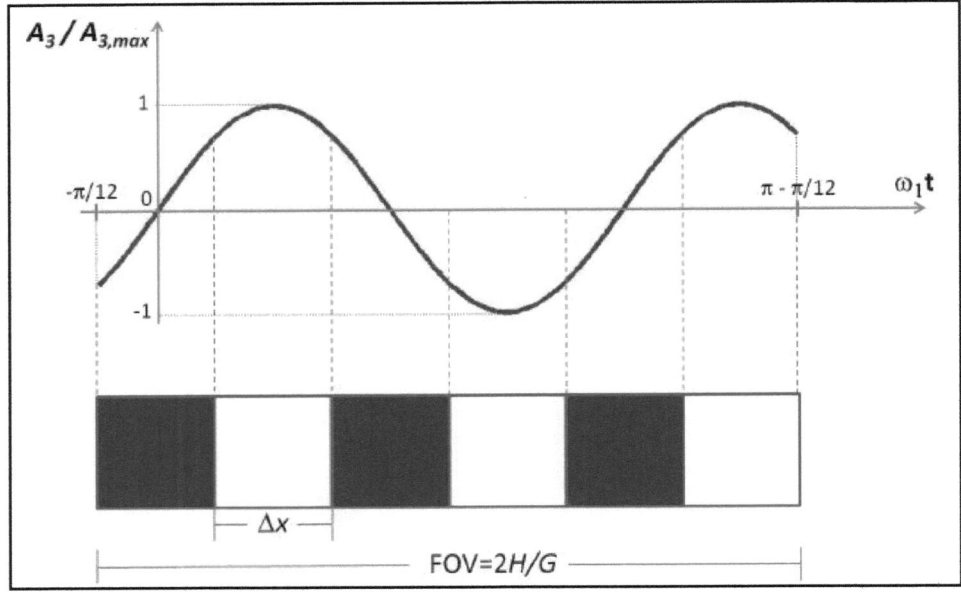

Fig. 1. Dependence between the imageable voxel length Δx and the field of view FOV for the 3rd Harmonic A_3. ω_1 is the frequency of the 1st Harmonic A_1. The abscissa runs from $-\pi/12$ to $\pi-\pi/12$ (for demonstration purposes shifted from zero), which equals a total range of $\Delta\omega_1 t = \pi$. To separate two neighbouring amounts of nanoparticles their corresponding voxels have to be distinguishable by a change of the signal. For the 3rd Harmonic this is possible using 6 voxels within the FOV meaning 3 voxels with signals at an extreme point (white squares) and 3 voxels with signals around zero (black squares).

Thus, taking voxel lengths, tracer concentration and MPI scanner noise level into account, the maximal number of detectable harmonics or the maximal FOV can be evaluated.

In order to demonstrate this framework experimentally at different drive field amplitudes, a serial dilution of Feraspin R® (nanoPET Pharma GmbH) was investigated by magnetic particle spectroscopy (MPS) using a commercial MPS spectrometer (Bruker Biospin).

Corresponding Author: F. Palmetshofer, florian.palmetshofer@ptb.de

The noise level of the spectrometer was defined as the standard deviation of the signal of an empty sample holder. The minimum detectable concentration of Feraspin R® was evaluated for the measurement volume of the MPS (30µl) and from there extrapolated to cubic MPI voxel volumes of 0.216µl (=0.6 x 0.6 x 0.6 mm³), 1.728 µl (=1.2 x 1.2 x 1.2 mm³) and 8 µl (=2 x 2 x 2 mm³).

For a concentration of 100 µmol/L the maximum number of detectable higher harmonics in MPS is limited to 19 and 29 for 5mT/µ0 and 10mT/µ0 drive field amplitude, respectively. Extrapolating to MPI voxel volume, the maximum number of detectable higher harmonics for field amplitudes of 5, 10, 18 and 25 mT/µ0 was found to be 3, 7, 9, 11 for a voxel volume of 0.216 µl, 11, 15, 27 and 35 for 1.728 µl and 15, 27, 41 and 55 for 8 µl, respectively. Applying the above mentioned formula, the possible FOV can be calculated from these results. Thus, it was shown that the principle helps to determine the maximum FOV for given tracer concentrations and voxel volume. Similarly the minimal voxel volume for a given FOV can be determined. This might be used as an application-oriented way of describing MPI tracers with respect to the noise level of a scanner device.

Acknowledgements: This work was supported by the German Federal Ministry of Economics and Technology grant No. KF2303711UW2. We thank nanoPET Pharma GmbH for providing Feraspin R®.

Corresponding Author: F. Palmetshofer, florian.palmetshofer@ptb.de

P32 OPTIMIZATION OF INHOMOGENEOUS EXCITATION FIELDS IN MAGNETORELAXOMETRY IMAGING OF MAGNETIC NANOPARTICLES

Daniel Baumgarten[1], Friedemann Braune[1,2], Roland Eichardt[1], Jens Haueisen[1]

[1]Institut fuer Biomedizinische Technik und Informatik, Technische Universität Ilmenau, Germany
[2]Abteilung Bildverarbeitung und Medizintechnik, Fraunhofer-Institut fuer Integrierte Schaltungen IIS, Erlangen, Germany

The distribution of magnetic nanoparticles can be quantitatively determined from multichannel magnetorelaxometry measurements by minimum norm estimation techniques [1]. It could be shown that the sequential activation of inhomogeneous excitation fields considerably enhances the imaging quality compared to homogeneous activation of the particles [2, 3]. In first studies, single coils were consecutively activated. We aim at further advancing this imaging technology by finding suitable activation patterns involving multiple excitation coils. In this paper, two approaches for finding optimal coil currents are presented. Figures-of-merit for this optimization are the spatial sensitivity and the condition of the underlying inverse problem that estimates the particle distribution from the relaxation measurements.

The first approach estimates currents that consecutively seek homogeneous spatial sensitivity. The sensitivity of a voxel in the source space describes its impact on the sensor system. It is influenced by the positions of voxels and sensors and by the excitation field in the respective voxel. Whereas the first is fixed within the given setup, the latter can be controlled by the currents in the excitation coils. By solving an inverse problem, currents are iteratively estimated to converge to a homogeneous sensitivity in the complete source space or in single planes thereof, respectively. Thus, it is ensured that all voxels contribute equally to the imaging. In the second approach, a particle swarm optimization (PSO) algorithm determines current parameters that minimize the condition number of the inverse problem The condition indicates the stability of the inverse solution regarding noise which considerably influences the imaging quality. In PSO, several sets of parameters (particles) are iteratively moved through the search space by updating them based on their own and the globally best value of a target function. In our application, one parameter set contains the parameters describing the currents for all coils and time samples and a minimum condition number value is searched.

Both approaches are investigated in simulation studies involving surrogate sensor and coil setups. Two-dimensional and three-dimensional particle distributions could be reconstructed. Seeking homogeneous sensitivity in the complete source space, the best imaging quality is achieved after activation with 5 excitation patterns and does not visibly improve thereafter. However, a fully homogeneous sensitivity is not achieved for the given setup. The given sensitivity is better approached in the plane-wise paradigm and better imaging results are obtained with the same number of excitation patterns than in the full 3D paradigm. For the second approach, starting from random initializations of the current parameters, our PSO algorithm considerably reduces the condition number and improves the imaging quality. Depending on the number of excitation patterns, appropriate parameters are obtained within a maximum of 80 iterations. Further iterations yield only marginal improvement.

Our results demonstrate the principal applicability of both approaches. The obtained activation patterns allow for a better imaging quality using a lower number of activation sequences compared to the conventional single coil activation. For the given setups, plane-wise sensitivity optimization yields the best imaging results among the presented approaches.

Corresponding Author: D. Baumgarten, daniel.baumgarten@tu-ilmenau.de

[1] D. Baumgarten, M. Liehr, F. Wiekhorst, U. Steinhoff, P. Muenster, P. Miethe, L. Trahms and J. Haueisen: Magnetic nanoparticle imaging by means of minimum norm estimates from remanence measurements. Med. Biol. Eng. Comp. 46, 2008, pp. 1177-1185.

[2] U. Steinhoff, F. Wiekhorst, D. Baumgarten, J. Haueisen and L. Trahms, Imaging of magnetic nanoparticles based on magnetorelaxometry with sequential activation of inhomogeneous magnetization fields. Biomed. Tech., 55:S1(A), 2010, pp. 22-25.

[3] G. Crevecoeur, D. Baumgarten, U. Steinhoff, J. Haueisen, L. Trahms and L. Dupré: Advancements in magnetic nanoparticle reconstruction using sequential activation of excitation coil arrays using magnetorelaxometry. IEEE Trans. Mag., 48:4, 2011 pp. 1313-1316.

Corresponding Author: D. Baumgarten, daniel.baumgarten@tu-ilmenau.de

P33 DUAL MODELS OF SCANNING SQUID BIOSUSCEPTOMETRY FOR SIMULTANEOUS FUNCTIONAL IMAGES OF MAGNETIC- NANOPARTICLES DISTRIBUTION AND STRUCTURAL IMAGES OF ANIMAL BODIES

H.E. Horng[1], J. J. Chieh[1], K. W. Huang[2], C. Y. Hong[3], H. C. Yang[4]

[1]Institute of Electro-Optical Science and Technology, National Taiwan Normal University, Taipei, Taiwan
[2]Department of Surgery & Hepatitis Research Center, National Taiwan University Hospital, Taipei, Taiwan
[3]Graduate Institute of Biomedical Engineering, National Chung Hsing University, Taichung, Taiwan
[4]Department of Electro-optical Engineering, Kun Shan University, Tainan, Taiwan

To image magnetic nanoparticles (MNPs) on animal bodies, physicians often use magnetic resonance imaging (MRI) to determine the superparamagetic characteristics of MNPs during preoperative analysis. However, MRI is unsuitable for other biomedical applications, such as the curative surgical resection of tumors or pharmacokinetic studies of MNPs, because of the requirement of nonmetal environments and high financial cost of frequent examination, respectively. Thus, researchers have proposed other nonmagnetic imaging technologies, such as fluorescence, using multimodal MNPs with nonmagnetic indicators. The development of a magnetic instrument based on the other magnetic characteristics of MNPs avoids the disadvantages of multimodal MNPs, including the biosafety risk. Based on the alternating current (AC) susceptibility of MNPs, previous research has demonstrated the magnetic examination of scanning superconducting-quantum-interference-device (SQUID) biosusceptometry (SSB). This study, using a low-noise charge-coupled-device (CCD) type of a video camera, reports the integration of SSB and CCD to immediately image the magnetic signals on animal bodies or organic tissue. This real-time imaging by SSB increases the usefulness of MNPs for more clinical applications, including the imaging-guided curative surgical resection of tumors.

Corresponding Author: H. E. Horng, phyfv001@scc.ntnu.edu.tw

P34 MAGNETIC PARTICLE IMAGING USING SECOND AND THIRD HARMONIC OF MAGNETIZATION RESPONSE

Hong-Chang Yang[1], Herng-Er Horng[2], Shu-Hsien Liao[2], Jen-Je Chieh[2]

[1]Department of Electro-optical Engineering, Kun Shan University, Tainan, Taiwan
[2]Institute of Electro-Optical Science and Technology, National Taiwan Normal University, Taipei, Taiwan

Magnetic particle imaging (MPI) is a new imaging technique which performs a direct measurement of the magnetization of magnetic nanoparticles. In this paper, we presented our 2-dimensional magnetic nanoparticle imaging system for detecting the second and third harmonic signal from magnetic nanoparticles. For second harmonic signal detection, the signal is generated from the magnetic nanoparticles under a bias magnetic field. For third harmonic signal detection, the signal is generated from the magnetic nanoparticles at field-free point. In our system we measure the second and third harmonic signal from the magnetization of magnetic nanoparticle at the same time and compare the imaging result from second and third harmonic signal. The imaging resolution included the concentration and the spatial resolution of MNPs is demonstrated by using our magnetic particle imaging system.

Corresponding Author: H.-C. Yang, hcyang@phys.ntu.edu.tw

P35 DC AND AC MAGNETIC SUSCEPTOMETRY OF SUPERPARAMAGNETIC FLUIDS AND FLIMS BY OPTICAL POLARIMETRY

Philipp Aebischer, Victor Lebedev, Antoine Weis

Department of Physics, University of Fribourg, Switzerland

We present a simple optical experiment for static (DC) and AC magnetic susceptibility measurements of superparamagnetic fluids and films. We demonstrate the technique by measuring the $B(H)$ dependence in static fields, from which we deduce the harmonic response of the samples to AC field excitation. The predicted AC response is confirmed by AC susceptibility measurements using the same apparatus. The application of an external magnetic field orients the magnetization vector of superparamagnetic iron oxide nanoparticles (SPIONs) along the field [1]. In granular solids this orientation is defined by Néel relaxation, while in colloidal suspensions both Néel and Brownian (rotational diffusion) relaxation contribute [2]. The $B(H)$ dependence of these superparamagnetic materials is described by a Langevin function, and the sample magnetization induces an optical anisotropy that can be detected by optical polarimetry [3] both in DC and AC measurements.

In our experiments we use the Faraday rotation of linearly polarized light to measure of the samples' magnetization. A scheme of the deployed apparatus is shown in Fig. 1a. A 780 nm diode laser beam traverses the sample exposed to either a static magnetic field H or a field of amplitude H_{RMS} oscillating at frequency n_{mod} produced by a solenoid. The Faraday rotation angle $\theta \propto B$ is measured by balanced photodetectors following a polarizing beam splitter (PBS) oriented at 45° with respect to the incident polarization. The differential signal is demodulated by a lock-in amplifier referenced to the chopper frequency n_{mod} for DC measurements or to odd harmonics $(2n+1)n_{mod}$ of the field modulation for AC measurements.

Figure 1b shows the experimentally recorded magnetization curve of an aqueous solution of 10 nm diameter magnetite particles (Ferrotec EMG 707), together with a Langevin function fit. The results of the harmonic response measurements are shown in Fig. 1c, together with the dependence predicted from the magnetization curve of Fig. 1b, similar to the treatment presented in Ref. [4]. We have further investigated the (modulation) frequency dependence of the linear susceptibility of liquid and dry samples. Results for the EMG 707 sample are shown in Fig. 1d, where the solid lines represent Lorentzian fits based on a model particle size distribution.

Results of measurements on other liquid and solid samples shall be presented at the conference.

We acknowledge financial support by Grant 200021_149542 of the Swiss National Science Foundation.

Corresponding Author: P. Aebischer, philipp.aebischer@unifr.ch

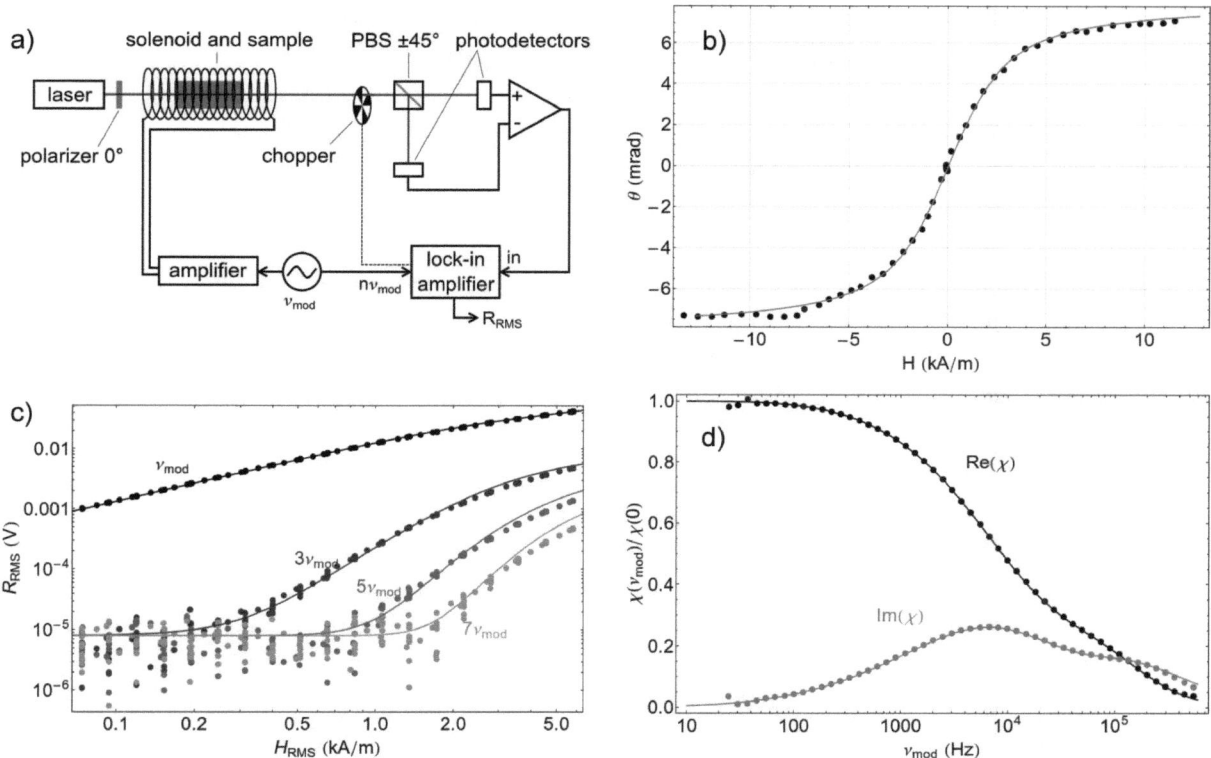

Figure 1: Optical measurements of AC/DC susceptibilities of a Ferrotec EMG 707 sample, diluted 1:500 in water: a: Optical polarimeter; b: Magnetization curve with Langevin function fit; c: Excitation amplitude dependence of harmonic response under AC (n_{mod} = 450 Hz) excitation; d: Frequency dependence of linear susceptibility, together with size distribution weighted Lorentzian fits.

[1] M. Knobel, W. C. Nunes, L. M. Socolovsky, E. De Biasi, J. M. Vargas, J. C. Denardin, "Superparamagnetism and Other Magnetic Features in Granular Materials: A Review on Ideal and Real Systems", J. Nanosci. Nanotechnol. 8, 2836 (2008)

[2] R. Kötitz, P. C. Fannin, L. Trahms, "Time domain study of Brownian and Néel relaxation in ferrofluids", J. Magn. Magn. Mater. 149, 42 (1995)

[3] S.-H. Chung, M. Grimsditch, A. Hoffmann, S. D. Bader, J. Xie, S. Peng, S. Sun, "Magneto-optic measurement of Brownian relaxation of magnetic nanoparticles", J. Magn. Magn. Mater. 320, 91 (2008)

[4] S. Vandendriessche, W. Brullot, D. Slavov, V. K. Valev, T. Verbiest, "Magneto-optical harmonic susceptometry of superparamagnetic materials", Appl. Phys. Lett. 102, 161903 (2013)

Corresponding Author: P. Aebischer, philipp.aebischer@unifr.ch

P36 SPATIALLY RESOLVED IN VITRO SPION MAGNETORELAXOMETRY USING ATOMIC MAGNETOMETERS

Victor Lebedev, Simone Colombo, Vladimir Dolgovskiy, Antoine Weis

Department of Physics, University of Fribourg, Switzerland

The spatially resolved quantitative detection of magnetic nano-tracers is a rapidly evolving field of research in material science and biomedical applications as well as in fundamental studies of magnetic material properties [1]. MPI (magnetic particle imaging) is one of the most powerful imaging techniques [2] for superparamagnetic nanoparticles (SPIONs). Its spatial encoding relies on the SPIONs' field dependent anharmonic response that is detected by magnetic pick-up.

Our imaging approach (Fig. 1a) deploys centimeter-sized magnetic field sensor based on atomic magnetometers [3] to image a two-dimensional projection of the field pattern produced by magnetized SPIONs, from which the field source distribution can, in principle, be reconstructed. The heart of the sensor is a cubic glass cell containing Cs vapor and a buffer gas, in which a thin sheet of light prepares an ensemble of quasi-immobilized spin-polarized atoms that act as field sensors. The atomic magnetization, stabilized by weak (<1mT) magnetic field is resonantly destroyed by magnetic resonance. The degree of magnetization is monitored via the resonance fluorescence emitted by the vapor (low intensity for large magnetization, and vice-versa). The magnetic field from the SPIONs shifts the magnetic resonance frequency, thereby altering the fluorescence yield. Field images are obtained by recording the fluorescence emitted by the cell with a CCD camera.

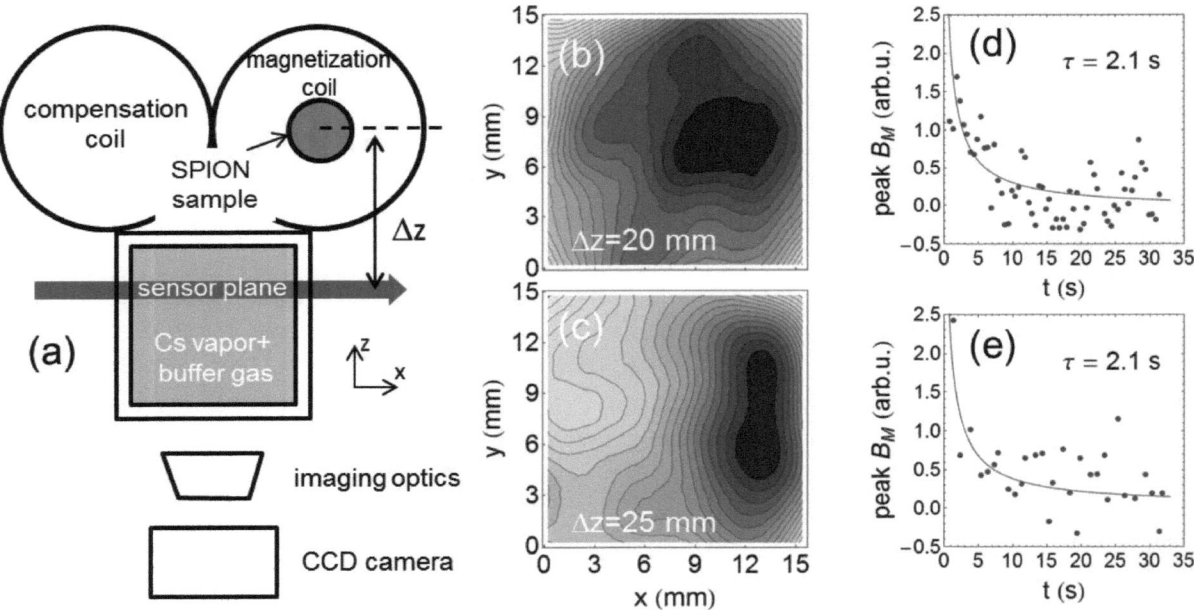

Figure 1: (a) Top view of the experimental set-up up for imaging MRX of SPIONs; (b,c) sample field maps at different sensor planes; (d,e) time evolution of the maximal field in (b,c), dots: experimental values, solid lines: fits of the form $A \ln(1 + \tau / t)$.

Here we demonstrate the method described above by recording the field distribution from a 2 mm high, 8 mm diameter matrix doped with 20 nm magnetite nanoparticle in a 15×15 mm² plane at different distances from the sample.

Corresponding Author: V. Lebedev, victor.lebedev@unifr.ch

The sample is magnetized in a 1 mT field for 20 seconds, after which we record 36 frames of the CCD camera, each exposed for 1 s. In an offline analysis the intensity of the last frame (reference image) is subtracted from all previous frames. Figures 1b,c show the first CCD frames, recorded 0.5 s after the end of the magnetization pulse. We have also performed a dynamic analysis of the data by extracting the peak magnetic field value in the time-dependent maps, yielding the results shown in Figs. 1d,e that exhibit the Néel relaxation of the sample's magnetization. We note that these early experimental results do not yet allow us a full quantitative interpretation. Work towards this goal is underway. By moving the illumination light sheet the method allows to access the third dimension of the field pattern, thereby easing source reconstruction. This method of spatially resolved magnetometry developed here is a relatively simple way to access full 3D field patterns. Based on the diffusion length of the sensor atoms in the buffer gas we estimate a sub-mm spatial resolution in the imaging plane. The accuracy of the method is limited by the design the of the magnetization coil. Sensitivity of the measurement is limited by the light detection sensitivity of the camera employed, and light source and magnetic environment stability. We see no major limitations for upscaling the sensor size to several cm, thus allowing the study of tissue samples and small organs/organisms.

We acknowledge financial support by Grant 200021_149542 of the Swiss National Science Foundation.

[1] Q.A. Pankhurst, J. Connolly, S.K. Jones, and J. Dobson, "Applications of magnetic nanoparticles in biomedicine", J. Phys. D: Appl. Phys. 36, 167 (2013).

[2] B. Gleich and J. Weizenecker, "Tomographic imaging using the nonlinear response of magnetic particles", Nature 435, 1214 (2005).

[3] D. Budker and M. Romalis, "Optical magnetometry", Nature Physics 3, 227 (2007)

Poster

Magnetic Nanoparticles & Tracer Materials

P37 TRACERS FOR MAGNETIC PARTICLE IMAGING CONSISTING OF AGGLOMERATED SINGLE CORES

Silvio Dutz[1], Norbert Buske[2], Norbert Löwa[3], Dietmar Eberbeck[3], Lutz Trahms[3]

[1]Ilmenau University of Technology, Institute of Biomedical Engineering and Informatics, Germany
[2]MagneticFluids, Berlin, Germany
[3]Physikalisch-Technische Bundesanstalt Berlin, Germany

Magnetic Particle Imaging (MPI) is a promising novel medical imaging technique allowing the background-free localization of magnetic nanoparticles (MNP) with high temporal and spatial resolution [1]. The properties of magnetic nanoparticles used as MPI tracer materials are of fundamental importance for resulting image quality [2]. At the moment the clinically approved MRI contrast agent Resovist® is the mostly used MNP sample for MPI. Measurements revealed that a minority of aggregates (consisting of primary crystallites) within the fluid is responsible for Resovist®'s preferential performance. Quite likely, this configuration is of crucial significance for MNP serving as MPI tracers. The present article reports on preparation and characterization of aqueous ferrofluids containing specially designed MNP to be used as tracers for MPI.

Following the example of Resovist®, clusters of small primary particles (so called magnetic multicore particles) were prepared. For this, a hydrosol of clustered *positively* charged magnetite nanoparticles without any organic components was fractionated by ultracentrifugation. The soft agglomerated MNP in the supernatant were used as an intermediate to subsequently prepare carboxymethylated dextran coated *negatively* charged clusters. Magnetic measurements (susceptometry, vibrating sample magnetometry, magnetic particle spectroscopy), transmission electron microscopy (TEM), dynamic light scattering (DLS), and X-ray diffraction (XRD) were used to characterize the obtained MNP regarding size, structure, and magnetic properties. Saturation magnetization Ms and size distribution of effective magnetic domain diameters (i.e. effective magnetic core size) were estimated from M(H) data, according to [3]. The measurements were performed with a commercial susceptometer (MPMS, Quantum Design). Additionally, the core size distribution (in terms of crystallite sizes) was obtained by analyzing the shape of the XRD intensity distribution by using an X-ray diffractometer (X'Pert Pro MPD). Furthermore, the hydrodynamic diameter of the MNP was measured by DLS using the Zetasizer 3000 (Malvern Instruments, UK). For all size distributions, spherical particles with diameters d obeying a log-nomal function $f(d)$ were assumed. Based on these considerations, the diameter of the mean volume d_V and the dispersion parameter σ were estimated. To evaluate the performance of the MNP as MPI tracer materials a magnetic particle spectrometer (MPS-3, Bruker) was used. In this study, all MPS measurements were performed at 25 mT magnetic field amplitude and an excitation frequency of 25 kHz.

The core sizes distribution parameters for the MNP hydrosol and the coated MNP estimated by XRD are d_V = 8.5 nm and 8.5 nm as well as σ = 0.36 and 0.37, respectively. Furthermore, the magnetic size distributions derived from M(H) data (d_V = 6.4 nm and 6.4 nm as well as σ = 0.537 and 0.531, respectively) are similar to those of the core size distributions from XRD. DLS of the samples results in hydrodynamic diameter of d_V = 97 nm for the MNP hydrosol and d_V = 109 nm for the coated MNP. Discrepancy of magnetic core size (M(H), XRD) and hydrodynamic diameter (DLS) confirms multicore structure. The prepared clusters show a size of nearly twice the diameter of aggregates found in Resovist® (d_V = 45 nm [4]). In contrast to Resovist®, neither for the core sizes nor for the magnetic sizes a bimodal distribution was found. The saturation magnetization Ms of the MNP hydrosol and the coated MNP, being 441 kA/m and 417 kA/m, respectively, were about 20% higher than for Resovist®.

Corresponding Author: S. Dutz, silvio.dutz@gmail.com

MPS signals of the investigated samples (normalized to their 3rd harmonic amplitude) are shown in Fig. 1. Investigated samples exhibit a MPS spectrum with similar initial slope as Resovist® but a steeper decay for higher harmonics. The absolute signal amplitudes, normalized to the respective iron content, were about 20% less than for Resovist® for the third harmonic and even less for higher harmonics. Compared to Feraheme® (a clinically approved formulation of small single core MNP) the here prepared clusters show higher MPS signal amplitudes until the 23rd harmonic and one order of magnitude higher when normalized to iron content.

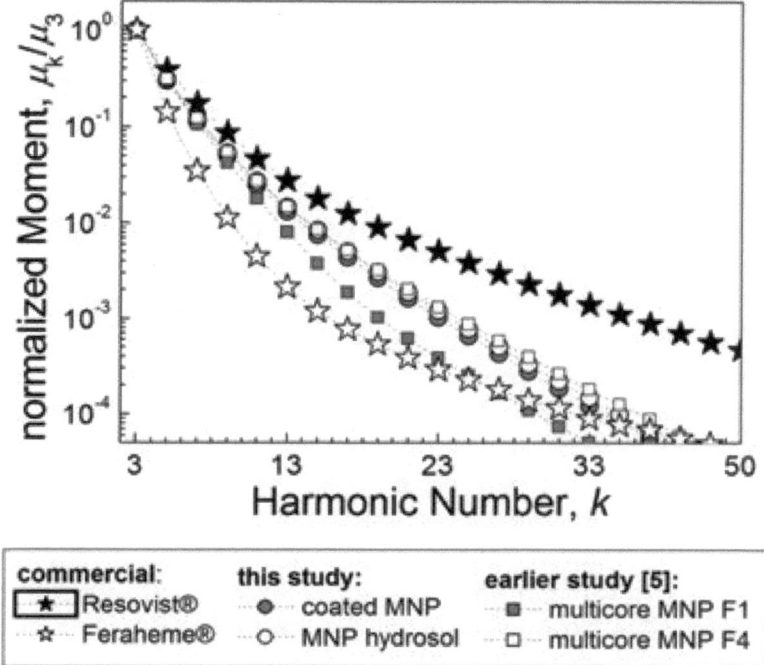

Figure 1: MPS measurement (25 mT, 25 kHz, results normalized to 3rd harmonic amplitude) of coated MNP (grey circles), MNP hydrosol (open circles) and the commercially available systems Resovist® (filled stars) and Feraheme® (open stars). For comparison, data for more compact multicore MNP (squares) of a previous study (prepared following a different route [5]) are shown.

As the measurement results show, clusters of small primary particles were prepared. Both, core size distribution and magnetic properties were not significantly influenced by the coating procedure. Compared to Resovist®, no second fraction of not clustered single cores could be identified from XRD and M(H) data. The MPS signals of the coated MNP and the MNP hydrosols were similar and in the order of Resovist® but exhibiting a steeper decay for higher harmonics. Probably, this problem can be solved by optimization of the packing density of the clusters - influencing exchange and dipole-dipole interactions between single cores by this way.

References

[1] B. Gleich, J. Weizenecker. *Nature* 435, 1214-17 (2005).

[2] R. M. Ferguson, A. P. Khandhar, K. Krishnan. *Appl. Phys.* 111, 07B318 (2012).

[3] D. Eberbeck, F. Wiekhorst, S. Wagner, L. Trahms. *Appl. Phys.* 98, 182502 (2011).

[4] D. Eberbeck, M. Kettering, C. Bergemann, P. Zirpel, I. Hilger, L. Trahms. *Appl. Phys.* 42, 405002 (2010).

[5] S. Dutz, D. Eberbeck, R. Müller, M. Zeisberger. In: Magnetic Particle Imaging, *Springer Proceedings in Physics* 140, 78-83 (2012).

Corresponding Author: S. Dutz, silvio.dutz@gmail.com

P38 FERROFLUIDS OF MODIFIED ULTRA SMALL MAGNETIC PARTICLES FOR APPLICATION IN THERANOSTICS

Norbert Buske[1], Natascha Schelero[2], Lars Dähne[2], Ines Krumbein[3], Jürgen R. Reichenbach[3], Silvio Dutz[4]

[1]MagneticFluids, Berlin, Germany
[2]Surflay Nanotec GmbH, Berlin, Germany
[3]University Hospital Jena, Center of Radiology, Institute for Diagnostic and Interventional Radiology I, Medical Physics Group, Germany
[4]Ilmenau University of Technology, Institute of Biomedical Engineering and Informatics, Germany

Multifunctional ferrofluids (FF) have great potential for being simultaneously used in diagnostics and therapy, also known as theranostics. As a typical example one can combine an imaging technique (MPI or MRI) for detection of cancer cells with therapy methods like drug targeting. For both applications the local particle and drug concentration at the target cells should be as high as possible to obtain a significant MPI/MRI signal and a high therapeutic effect. In our study two different strategies were applied to improve the local particle concentration in tissue: (A) Exploiting the long half life time of ultra small superparamagnetic iron oxide (USPIO) particles in the blood circulation (up to 10h), which enables a long contact time of the particles towards the target cells and (B) Creating an antigen-antibody interaction to the target cells by modifying the USPIO particle's surface with specific antibodies. USPIO carboxymethylated dextran (CMD) magnetite particle FF were prepared in an one step process by aqueous co-precipitation in the presence of CMD excess and further dialysis and filtering processes. Additionally, a combined centrifugation-dialysis process was used for FF purification and enrichment of the particle concentration up to 10 mg_{Fe}/ml. The as prepared aggregation stable USPIO-FFs were coated first with streptavidin followed by biotinylated specific anti-bodies to establish an antigen-antibody fixing. The hydrodynamic size, polydispersity index, and zeta-potential of the USPIO-CMD-FF were measured by dynamic light scattering (DLS). The core size was determined by transmission electron microscopy (TEM), vibrating sample magnetometry (VSM) magnetization curves, and X-ray diffraction (XRD). The amount of coupled and active streptavidin was determined by quantitative analysis of fluorescein-biotin coupling to the FF particles. MPI performance was tested by MPS measurements at 25 mT and 25 kHz and MRI relaxation times were determined at 1.5 T for different USPIO concentrations. A superparamagnetic behavior of the particles was confirmed by negligible coercivity and a relative remanence of 0.02. The hydrodynamic diameter from DLS is on the order of 20 to 30 nm. Core size was determined to be 5 to 7 nm. The particles are suitable as MPI tracers as well as contrast agents for MRI. In the presentation the imaging performance of these USPIO-FF as well as antibody coupling will be discussed in more detail. Here prepared multifunctional, in vivo applicable USPIO-CMD-FFs modified with antibodies are potential candidates for application in theranostics by combining imaging with drug targeting.

Acknowledgements: The presented work was supported in the framework of the NIMINI-project No.: 01EZ0815. The USPIO-FFs were prepared at Capsulution AG, Berlin and the antibody surface coating was performed at Surflay-Nanotec, Berlin. MPS experiments were carried out by Norbert Löwa, PTB Berlin.

Corresponding Author: N. Buske, n.buske@magneticfluids.de

P39 BACTERIAL MAGNETOSOMES AS A NEW TYPE OF BIOGENIC MPI TRACERS

Alexander Kraupner[1], David Heinke[1], Rene Uebe[2], Dietmar Eberbeck[3], Nicole Gehrke[1], Dirk Schueler[2], Andreas Briel[1]

[1]nanoPET Pharma GmbH, Berlin, Germany
[2]Ludwig-Maximilians-Universität, Planegg-Martinsried, Germany
[3]Physikalisch-Technische Bundesanstalt, Berlin, Germany

Biomineralization is the process whereby minerals are formed by living organisms to form features such as teeth and bones, spicules and nacre produced by humans, sponges and some mollusks, respectively. The purpose of the biomineral is dependent on the organism but is known to serve a protective or structural function. Biominerals exhibit extraordinary material properties such as the combination of extreme mechanical robustness and extreme lightweight as in the case of nacre. Another amazing example are so-called magnetosomes, membrane-enclosed iron oxide nanoparticles biomineralized by magnetotactic bacteria as magnetic sensor for magnetotaxis, which is the orientation along the earth's magnetic field.[1] Such magnetosomes are characterized by distinctive monodispersity in size and shape and consist of a monocrystalline magnetite phase- all features, which are intensively pursued but only partially achieved by the synthesis of iron oxide nanoparticles in the lab.

Magnetic Particle Imaging (MPI) is a new and promising imaging technology that requires the use of a magnetic tracer material. Although significant efforts have been undertaken to synthesize suitable MPI tracers and to understand their structure-efficacy relation, no ideal tracer exists to date. Different theories and approaches exist, involving iron oxide nanoparticles comprising, on the one hand, cores of crystal clusters[2] and, on the other hand, monocrystalline cores of large size[3]. Due to their significant crystal size (mature particles can grow up to 120 nm), high crystallinity and monodispersity, magnetosomes are promising candidates as novel MPI tracers.

Here, we present the investigation of magnetosomes isolated from the bacterium *Magnetospirillum gryphiswaldense* in relation to their MPI performance and in comparison to the current gold-standard, Resovist®. The wild-type as well as mutants of the magnetosomes with different particle sizes are investigated, which offer the possibility of size-dependent studies. In addition, we characterize the magnetic properties (MRX, M(H)) and the morphology of the particles by means of TEM, SAED and DLS.

We show that the MPS signal generated by the magnetosomes is highly improved compared to Resovist, although the magnetosomes are not perfectly monodisperse and uniform in shape. Furthermore, we observe a size-dependence of the MPS signal with the highest signal for the largest particles. Static magnetization curves show a significant higher susceptibility of the magnetosomes compared to Resovist, which allows first indications for the improved MPI performance. Although technical applications of magnetosomes have been hampered due to their technically challenging bioproduction, our contribution proves their potential as tracers and may stimulate new research efforts to synthesize such particles in the lab by biological and biomimetic synthetic routes.[4]

Corresponding Author: A. Kraupner, alexander.kraupner@nanopet.de

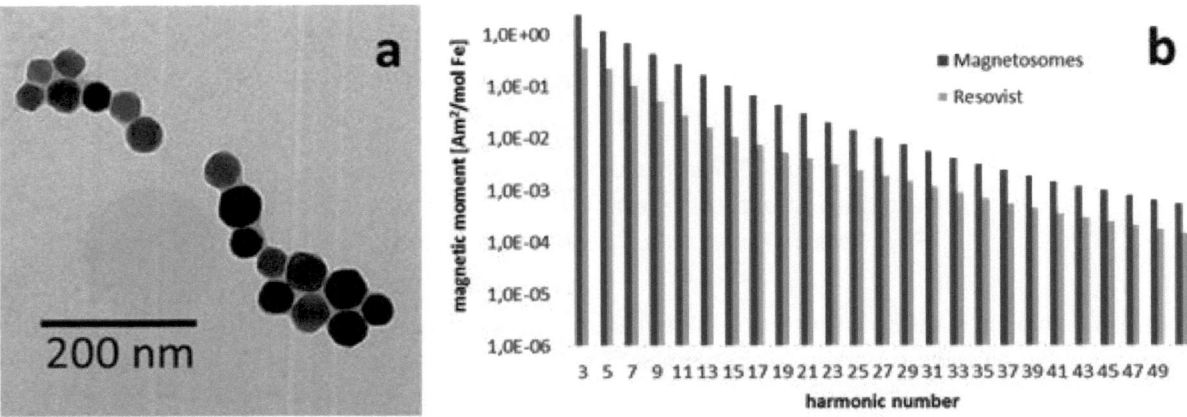

Fig. 1: a) TEM image of the magnetosomes and b) MPS spectrum measured at 25 mT/µ0 and 25.25 kHz

[1] Faivre, D., Schüler, D., Magnetotactic bacteria and magnetosomes, Chemical Reviews, 108(11), 4875-4898, 2008

[2] Gehrke, N. et al , New Perspectives for MPI: A Toolbox for Tracer Research, Magnetic Particle Imaging, T. M. Buzug and J. Borgert, Eds., Springer Proceedings in Physics, 140, 99-103, 2012

[3] Gleich, B., Weizenecker, J., Tomographic imaging using the nonlinear response of magnetic particles, Nature, 435(7046), 1214-1217, 2005

[4] Baumgartner, J. et al, Formation of Magnetite Nanoparticles at Low Temperature: From Superparamagnetic to Stable Single Domain Particles, Plos One, 8(3), e57070, 2013

Acknowledgements: This work was supported by the FP 7 of the European Union (NMP4-SL-2011-245542-Bio2MaN4MRI).

Corresponding Author: A. Kraupner, alexander.kraupner@nanopet.de

P40 THE IMPACT OF THE SIZE DISTRIBUTION OF NANOPARTICLES IN MAGNETIC NANOTHERMOMETRY

Zhongzhou Du, Wenzhong Liu, Jing Zhong, Paulo Cesar Morais

School of Automation, Huazhong University of Science and Technology, Wuhan, China

In recent years the material platform base on biocompatible magnetic nanoparticles has attracted increasing attention while addressing magnetic hyperthermia, magnetic particle imaging, and nanothermometry [1-4]. In these regards engineering of magnetic nanoparticles is of great significance to the new technologies performance. This study aims to evaluate the impact of the magnetic particle size distribution upon the accuracy of the temperature estimation while using AC magnetic fields to assess the information. Here, we focused on the standard deviation of the magnetic particle size distribution (δ) dependence of temperature estimation accuracy. According to the standard description of superparamagnetism using the first-order Langevin's function, the frequency spectrum of the magnetization is sensitive to the temperature [5]. Therefore, the harmonic amplitude of AC magnetization allows temperature estimation. In the present study, the temperature estimation is obtained by recording the harmonic amplitudes of the AC magnetization at different temperatures. Fig. 1 shows the temperature estimation errors for different standard deviation (δ) values. In the range of our investigation the maximum error we found for temperature estimation was about 1.08 K, with a temperature standard deviation of 0.8 K, when δ is 0.3 (log-normal distribution profile). In contrast, when we set δ equals to 0.2 nm we found the error for temperature estimation of about 0.14 K, with a standard deviation of 0.09 K. Our findings indicate that the temperature estimation error increases monotonically with δ. As δ decreases from 0.3 to 0.2, the temperature estimation accuracy increases nearly by a factor of 8. In conclusion, magnetic nanoparticle temperature estimation with higher accuracy is achieved by reducing the nanoparticle polydispersity.

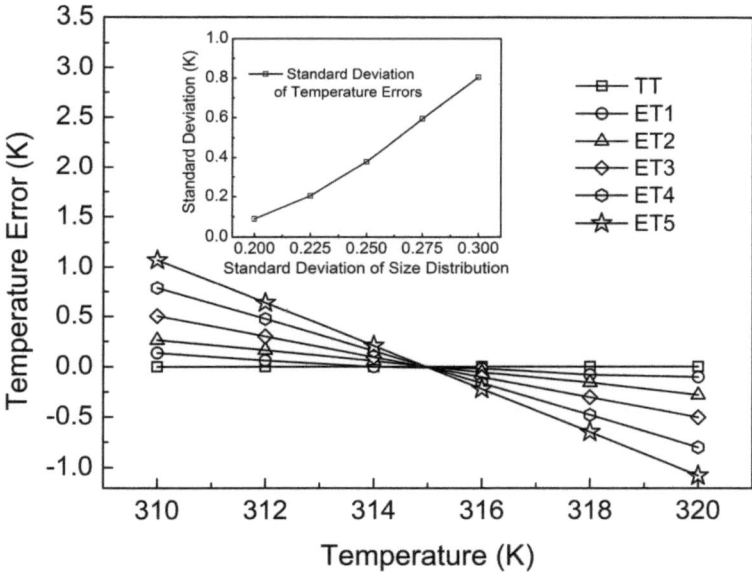

Fig. 1. Temperature probing error for different standard deviations of particle size distribution. ET1-ET5 represent the temperature errors for standard deviations of 0.200, 0.225, 0.250, 0.275 and 0.300 for average particle diameter of 2.4 nm. TT represents theoretical temperature. The inset shows the standard deviation of temperature estimated errors. The amplitude of AC applied field and the SNR of AC magnetization were set at 20 Oe and 100 dB, respectively.

Corresponding Author: J. Zhong, jingzhong@hust.edu.cn

[1] Chun-Han Hou, Sheng-Mou Hou, Yu-Sheng Hsueh, Jinn Lin, Hsi-Chin Wu, Feng-Huei Lin, The in vivo performance of biomagnetic hydroxyapatite nanoparticles in cancer hyperthermia therapy, Biomaterials, 30, 3956 (2009).

[2] B. Gleich and J. Weizenecker, Tomographic imaging using the nonlinear response of magnetic particles, Nature, 435, 1214 (2005).

[3] G. Kucsko, P. C. Maurer, N. Y. Yao, M. Kubo, H. J. Noh, P. K. Lo, H. Park, and M. D. Lukin, Nanometre-scale thermometry in a living cell. Nature, 500, 54 (2013).

[4] Jing Zhong, Wenzhong Liu, Zhongzhou Du, Paulo césar de Morais, Qing Xiang and Qingguo Xie, A noninvasive, remote and precise method for temperature and concentration estimation using magnetic nanoparticles, Nanotechnology, 23, 075703 (2012).

[5] Jing Zhong, Wenzhong Liu, Ming Zhou and Pu Zhang, Magnetic nanoparticle temperature estimation using AC magnetic field, Proceedings of IWMPI, Berkeley, United States, 2013, 978-1-4673-5522-3/13.

Corresponding Author: J. Zhong, jingzhong@hust.edu.cn

P41 AC MAGNETIZATION SPECTRUM FOR MAGNETIC NANOPARTICLE TEMPERATURE ESTIMATION: AN INVESTIGATION OF AC APPLIED MAGNETIC FIELD

Zhongzhou Du, Wenzhong Liu, Jing Zhong, Ming Zhou

School of Automation, Huazhong University of Science and Technology, Wuhan, China

Magnetic nanoparticle temperature estimation by AC magnetization spectrum is a novel, precise and non-invasive temperature measurement approach [1, 2]. AC applied magnetic field is one of important impact factors that leading to temperature error [3, 4]. In this report, the model for the minimum temperature estimation error in different AC applied magnetic field is simulated for specific magnetic nanoparticles. In the process of discretization for Langevin function, truncation error caused by the finite polynomial approximation method is found to be increased under an increasing AC field. Whereas, the relative error caused by random noise would decrease under an increasing AC field. So the estimated error decreases along with an increased AC field till the error reaches its minimum. And then the error increased with large field. Simulations (Fig.1) show that the total temperature estimation error varies with the AC field under the same SNR. When AC strength is less than 50Guass, random noise is a main contributor for estimation error. The total error reaches its minimum, with an AC field in between 150Guass to 200Guass. While field is above 250Gauss, the truncation error caused by finite polynomial approximation contributes the main error of temperature estimation. In summary, we find by simulation that temperature estimation error reach its minimum when AC field fall in 150Guass to 200Guass results.

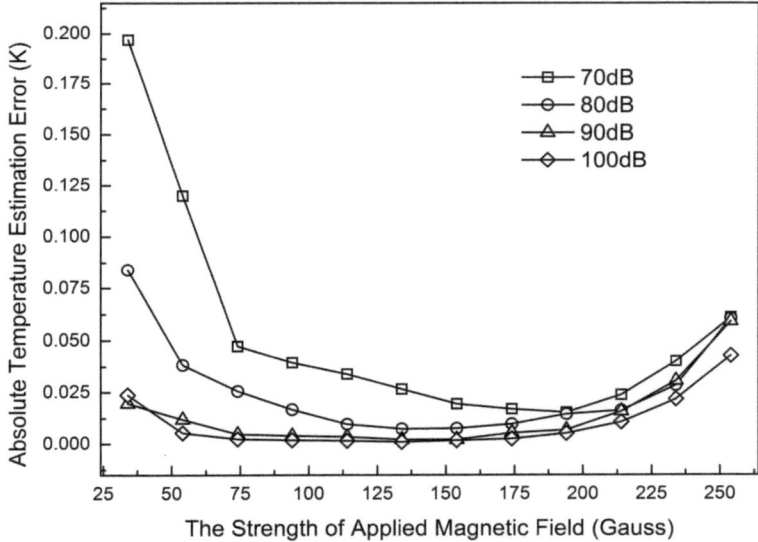

Fig.1. The temperature estimation errors in different AC magnetic fields with the same frequency of 105 Hz. The amplitude of AC magnetic fields is from 34 Gauss to 254 Gauss with a step of 20 Gauss. The effective magnetic moment is 2×10^{-19} emu.

Corresponding Author: W. Liu, lwz7410@hust.edu.cn

[1] John B. Weaver, Adam M. Rauwerdink and Eric W. Hansen, Magnetic nanoparticle temperature estimation, Medical Physics, 36, 1822 (2009).

[2] Jing Zhong, Wenzhong Liu, Zhongzhou Du, Paulo césar de Morais, Qing Xiang and Qingguo Xie, A noninvasive, remote and precise method for temperature and concentration estimation using magnetic nanoparticles, Nanotechnology, 23, 075703 (2012).

[3] Yin Li, Wenzhong Liu and Jing Zhong, Comparison of noninvasive and remote temperature estimation employing magnetic nanoparticles in DC and AC applied fields, Proceedings of I2MTC, Graz, Austria, 2012, 2738-2741.

[4] Jing Zhong, Wenzhong Liu, Ming Zhou and Pu Zhang, Magnetic nanoparticle temperature estimation using AC magnetic field, Proceedings of IWMPI, Berkeley, United States, 2013, 978-1-4673-5522-3/13.

Corresponding Author: W. Liu, lwz7410@hust.edu.cn

P42 COMPARISON OF TEMPERATURE ESTIMATION EMPLOYING MAGNETIZATION AND INVERSE SUSCEPTIBILITY OF MAGNETIC NANOPARTICLES IN DC FIELD

Ling Jiang, Wenzhong Liu, Jing Zhong

School of Automation, Huazhong University of Science and Technology, Wuhan, China

Design of noninvasive nanoscale thermometer with a high accuracy is a challenging research topic. In recent decades, several nanoscale thermometers have been developed employing the physical properties of nano-materials [1-3]. Magnetization and susceptibility, which are fundamental physical properties of magnetic nanoparticles, are capable of designing a nanoscale thermometer due to their temperature-sensitivity. In our previous studies, a nanoscale thermometer using inverse susceptibility of magnetic nanoparticles has been theoretically and experimentally investigated [3]. In this paper, both magnetization and inverse susceptibility of magnetic nanoparticles are utilized to estimate temperature in DC field by simulation, and their measurement accuracy was compared. Figure 1 shows the measured temperature using magnetization and inverse susceptibility as well as the measurement errors by 5th expansion order of Langevin function [4, 5]. With a SNR of 80dB, the maximum error in temperature estimation employing magnetization is about 0.36 K with a standard deviation of 0.26 K, lower than that for the measurement error employing inverse susceptibility which is about 1.66 K with a standard deviation of 0.92 K. This indicates that temperature estimation using magnetization is more accurate by a factor of about 4 than that using inverse susceptibility.

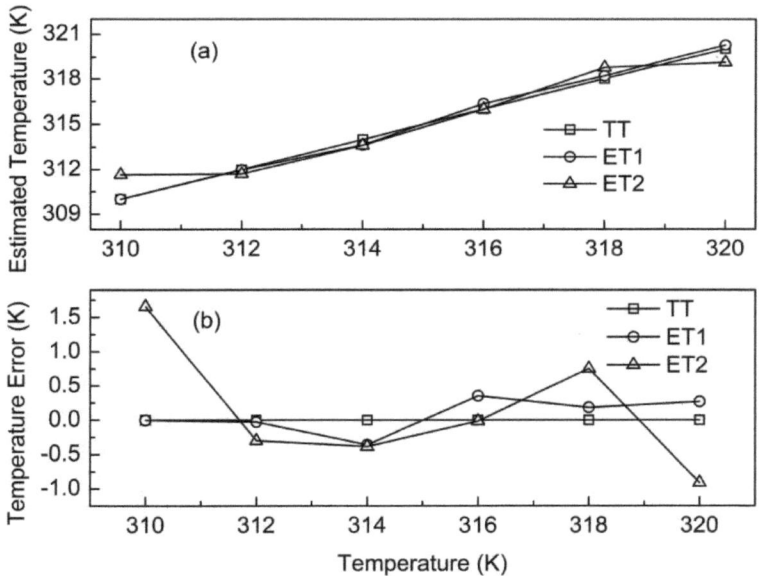

Fig. 1. ET1-ET2 in (a) represent estimated temperature by using magnetization and inverse susceptibility of magnetic nanoparticles at SNR of 80dB, while (b) shows the relevant temperature error. The applied magnetic fields are from 10 Gauss to 200 Gauss with a step of 10 Gauss. And the effective magnetic moment is 1×10^{-19} emu.

Corresponding Author: W. Liu, lwz7410@hust.edu.cn

[1] G. Kucsko, P. C. Maurer, N. Y. Yao, M. Kubo, H. J. Noh, P. K. Lo, H. Park, and M. D. Lukin, Nanometre-scale thermometry in a living cell, Nature, 500, 54 (2013).

[2] Fangmao Ye, Changfeng Wu, Yuhui Jin, Yang-Hsiang Chan, Xuanjun Zhang, and Daniel T. Chiu, Ratiometric Temperature Sensing with Semiconducting Polymer Dots, Journal of the American Chemical Society, 133, 8146 (2011).

[3] Jing Zhong, Wenzhong Liu, Zhongzhou Du, Paulo césar de Morais, Qing Xiang and Qingguo Xie, A noninvasive, remote and precise method for temperature and concentration estimation using magnetic nanoparticles, Nanotechnology, 23, 075703 (2012).

[4] Jing Zhong, Wenzhong Liu, Shiqiang Pi and Pu Zhang, Optimization for temperature estimation using magnetic nanoparticle: a set of equations solving solution investigation, Proceedings of I2MTC, Minneapolis, Unite States, 2013, 1329-1331.

[5] Yin Li, Wenzhong Liu and Jing Zhong, Comparison of noninvasive and remote temperature estimation employing magnetic nanoparticles in DC and AC applied fields, Proceedings of I2MTC, Graz, Austria, 2012, 2738-2741.

Corresponding Author: W. Liu, lwz7410@hust.edu.cn

P43 CONTINUOUSLY MANUFACTURED MAGNETIC POLYMERSOMES AS POTENTIAL THERANOSTIC TOOLS IN NANOMEDICINE

Regina Bleul[1], Norbert Löwa[2], Raphael Thiermann[3], Urs O. Häfeli[4], Gernot U. Marten[4], Michael J. House[5], Timothy G. St. Pierre[5], Lutz Trahms[2], Michael Maskos[6]

[1]Federal Institute for Materials Research and Testing, Berlin, Germany
[2]Physikalisch-Technische Bundesanstalt, Berlin, Germany
[3]Institut für physikalische Chemie, Johannes Gutenberg-Universität, Mainz, Germany
[4]Faculty of Pharmaceutical Sciences, University of British Columbia, Vancouver, Canada
[5]School of Physics, The University of Western Australia, Crawley, Australia
[6]Institut für Mikrotechnik Mainz GmbH, Germany

Systems for combined diagnostic and therapeutic approaches, so called theranostics, have gained the interest of many researchers because of their immense potential for directly monitoring therapy. Here, we present magnetic and drug loaded polymeric vesicles (polymersomes) as traceable drug carriers. Magnetic particle imaging (MPI) as a powerful imaging technique with its high sensitivity and spatial resolution may allow tracking of these magnetic nanotransporters inside the body. Micromixing technology as reliably controllable straightforward preparation method was used to manufacture drug-loaded magnetic polymersomes. The polymersomes are based on the FDA-approved triblock copolymer poly(ethylene oxide)-b-poly(propylene oxide)-b-poly(ethylene oxide). The anti-cancer drug camptothecin as well as magnetic nanoparticles (MNP) were loaded in situ during the polymersome formation. Successful incorporation of the MNP was confirmed by transmission electron microscopy. Dynamic light scattering measurements showed a relatively narrow size distribution of the hybrid polymersomes. Their stability in presence of serum proteins was also demonstrated by multi-angle light scattering. Camptothecin polymersomes reduced the cell viability of prostate cancer cells (PC-3) measured after 72 h significantly, while drug-free polymersomes showed no cytotoxic effects. Specific cell targeting to prostate cancer cells of bombesin-functionalized hybrid polymersomes was shown by flow cytometry and confocal microscopy.[1] Relaxometry measurements clearly demonstrated the capacity of magnetic polymersomes to generate significant T2-weighted MRI contrast. In vivo studies concerning the biodistribution profile and the in vivo MR contrast properties are in progress. First investigations of the performance of the magnetic polymersomes for MPI have shown promising results. Magnetic particle spectroscopy revealed that the absolute signal amplitudes, normalized to the respective iron content, were generally higher for the magnetic polymersomes than for Endorem® and Feraheme®. Even compared to Resovist® the signal amplitudes were only 50% less for the third harmonic. The encapsulated MNP in the polymersomes' membrane have a core diameter of about 10 nm and are not optimized for MPI. Thus, there is room for improvement in MPI performance, which is subject of ongoing work.

Continuously manufactured magnetic polymersomes that allow for direct monitoring of the biodistribution will be a further step from basic research towards the development of theranostic drug devices.

Corresponding Author: R. Bleul, regina.bleul@bam.de

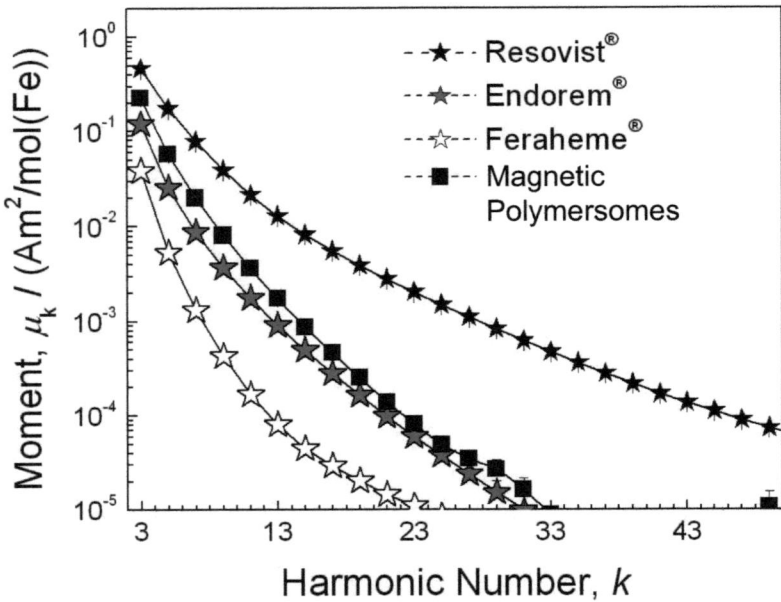

Figure 1 Magnetic particle spectroscopy: Signal spectrum of magnetic polymersomes compared to commercial contrast agents

[1] Bleul, R. et al. Continuously manufactured magnetic polymersomes - a versatile tool (not only) for targeted cancer therapy. Nanoscale 5, 11385-11393 (2013).

Corresponding Author: R. Bleul, regina.bleul@bam.de

P44 EVALUATION OF HYSTERESIS LOOP AND MAGNETIC RELAXATION TIME OF MAGNETIC NANOPARTICLES UNDER ALTERNATING MAGNETIC FIELD

Satoshi Ota[1], Kosuke Nakamura[1], Asahi Tomitaka[2], Tsutomu Yamada[1], Yasushi Takemura[1]

[1]Department of Electrical and Computer Engineering, Yokohama National University, Japan
[2]Department of Materials Science and Engineering, University of Washington, Seattle, USA

Superparamagnetic nanoparticles are used as an imaging agent. Magnetic particle imaging (MPI) is applicable to not only diagnostics but therapy such as hyperthermia and drug delivery. Integrative therapeutic and diagnostic application is called as theranostics. In particular, magnetic relaxation is one of the most important factors for both imaging and hyperthermia treatment. The evaluation of magnetic relaxation property is necessary to design the materials and instrument applying an external magnetic field. Magnetic relaxation is characterized by two distinct modes. Brownian relaxation is occurred by rotation of the particles. Néel relaxation is induced by rotation of the magnetic moment. The mechanism of magnetic relaxation is influenced by the primary and secondary size of magnetic nanoparticles, surface coating agent, state of materials, viscosity of medium. In this study, the magnetic relaxation properties of Resovist and other commercial magnetic nanoparticles were measured at frequency of several kiro heltz up to 500 kHz and high magnetic field up to 50 Oe. The commercial iron oxide nanoparticles of both of superparamagnetic and ferrimagnetic features were used for the measurements. The hysteresis loop under an applied alternating magnetic field was measured for estimating magnetic loss and effective magnetic relaxation time. The materials were prepared in powder form, dispersed state in medium, or fixed state by agarose / epoxy bond. Magnetic nanoparticles dispersed in medium were rotated by an alternating magnetic field, and both Brownian and Néel relaxation could occur. In contrast, fixation regulated rotation of the particles and only Néel relaxation could occur. Therefore, hysteresis loop of alternating magnetic field in dispersed and fixed samples directly indicated the magnetic relaxation mechanisms of measured materials. The dependency of area of the hysteresis loop on the frequency of magnetic field indicated the effective frequency of Brownian and Néel relaxation. Relaxation time was also calculated. Experimental estimation of effective relaxation time confirms the influence of size distribution, concentration, state, surface coating agent and medium. Thus, evaluation of magnetic loss and magnetic relaxation time measured under the alternating field condition which is used for MPI is the effective method to evaluate the mechanisms of magnetic relaxation and optimum material property.

Corresponding Author: S. Ota, ota-satoshi-gw@ynu.ac.jp

P45 DRIVE FIELD FREQUENCY DEPENDENT MPI PERFORMANCE OF SINGLE CORE MAGNETITE NANOPARTICLES

Christian Kuhlmann[1], Amit P. Khandhar[2], R. Matthew Ferguson[3], Scott J. Kemp[3], Kannan M. Krishnan[2], Thilo Wawrzik[1], Meinhard Schilling[1], Frank Ludwig[1]

[1]Institut fuer Elektrische Messtechnik und Grundlagen der Elektrotechnik, Technische Universität Braunschweig, Germany
[2]Department of Materials Science and Engineering, University of Washington, USA
[3]LodeSpin Labs, Washington, USA

The drive field frequency of Magnetic Particle Imaging (MPI) systems plays an important role for system design, safety requirements and tracer selection.

Because the commonly utilized MPI drive field frequency of 25 kHz might be increased in future system generations to avoid peripheral nerve stimulation, a performance evaluation of tracers at higher frequencies is desirable. In addition, the investigation of the drive-field-frequency dependence of the harmonic spectrum is beneficial for the development of proper models and thus helps to better understand particle properties.

We have studied magnetite nanoparticles that were optimized for MPI applications, utilizing Magnetic Particle Spectrometers (MPS) with drive field frequencies in the range from 1 kHz up to 100 kHz. The particles have core diameters of 25 nm from TEM measurements (25.3 from fitting to $M(H)$ data assuming a single log-normal distribution with geometric standard deviation of 0.23) and a hydrodynamic size of 77 nm (determined by dynamic light scattering). MPS measurements between 1 kHz and 10 kHz were performed with our spectrometer described in [1] whereas spectra in the frequency range above 10 kHz were recorded with a newly designed MPS system allowing one to adjust discrete drive frequencies of 10 kHz, 25 kHz, 50 kHz, and 100 kHz with rms amplitudes up to 25 mT. Optionally, additional static magnetic fields can be applied. In both MPS systems, gradiometric detection coils are utilized.

Immobilized particles were prepared from aqueous solutions by freeze-drying the sample in a mannitol matrix. Since the Brownian mechanism is blocked in this process, it allows one to study the frequency dependence of the Néel contribution. In order to exclude possible particle interactions, samples of different concentrations were characterized and compared.

Fig. 1 depicts MPS spectra measured for various drive-field frequencies between 1 kHz and 100 kHz at a rms field amplitude of 25 mT on a sample suspension and on an immobilized reference sample. As can be seen the spectral magnitude of the 3rd harmonic increases with drive frequency as a consequence of the induction law. On the other hand, the slope of the harmonic decay rises with increasing drive field frequency. The effect can be seen for mobile as well as immobile samples and is monotonous over the covered frequency range.

Immobilized particles show a significantly decreased signal and a steeper harmonic decay compared to mobile samples due to the large Néel time constant of the examined single-core particles.

Whereas the spectral magnitudes of the 3rd harmonic significantly differ for drive-field frequencies between 1 kHz and 10 kHz, the differences are only weak between 25 kHz and 100 kHz. Thus, the signal gain due to the induction law is partially compensated by the fact that most of the particles can no longer follow the fast drive field. This is supported by measurements of the ac susceptibility.

The observed drive-field-frequency dependence of the harmonic spectra will be compared to several models. Implications for the application of the examined particles as tracers for MPI at increased drive field frequencies and mitigation of the observed effects by the use of induction coils as sensors will be discussed.

Corresponding Author: C. Kuhlmann, c.kuhlmann@tu-bs.de

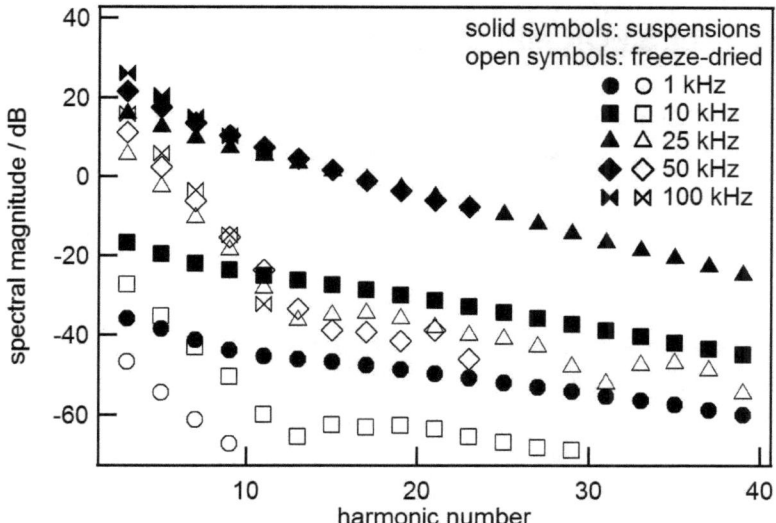

Fig. 1: Spectral magnitude versus harmonic number measured on suspension and immobilized reference samples normalized to same iron content for drive-field frequencies between 1 kHz and 100 kHz.

This work was supported by the German Federal Ministry of Economics and Technology under grant no. FKZ KF3061201UW2. APK, RMF, SK, KMK acknowledge support from the National Institutes of Health grant no. 2R42EB013520-02A1

[1]   T. Wawrzik, F. Ludwig, and M. Schilling, AIP Conf. Proc. 1311, 267 (2010)

Corresponding Author: C. Kuhlmann, c.kuhlmann@tu-bs.de

P46 STRUCTURAL CHARACTERIZATION OF CLUSTERED CORE IRON OXIDE NANOPARTICLES FOR MPI BY SMALL ANGLE X-RAY SCATTERING

Nicole Gehrke[1], Stefan Wellert[2], David Heinke[1], Andreas Briel[1], Dietmar Eberbeck[3]

[1]nanoPET Pharma GmbH, Berlin, Germany
[2]Stranski Laboratory, TU Berlin, Germany
[3]Bioelectricity and Biomagnetism, Physikalisch-Technische Bundesanstalt, Berlin, Germany

Iron oxide nanoparticles are the most promising MPI tracer candidates, but the relation between their structure and their MPI efficacy is still not understood. This is especially valid for such particles having iron oxide cores composed of clustered crystallites (so called multicore particles) which were observed to show unexpectedly high MPS amplitudes.

Small angle X-ray scattering (SAXS) is as an ideal tool for the investigation of nanostructures such as nanoparticles in bulk or solution[1]. Based on the sensitivity of X-rays on the electron density difference between sample and solvent elastically scattered X-ray radiation provides information about the structure and the length scales of the sample. Because standard SAXS allows the investigation of length scales between a few nanometers up to about 100 nanometers it is ideally suited to study this clustered core particle type and to provide information on the structure of the core as a whole as well as it`s sub-structure.

Here, we present a study involving the structural analysis of different in-house synthesized iron oxide nanoparticles of the clustered core type by means of SAXS. Although in terms of hydrodynamic size, crystallite size and coating material some of those particles exhibited very similar structures, they showed huge differences in their MPS efficacies[2].

The particle solutions were measured using a Kratky-camera system equipped with a sealed tube microsource. Initial data treatment and desmearing was done using the Saxsquant software package provided.

For all particles of this study we identified at least two length-scales in the SAXS curves: The range of low values of the scattering vector q was characteristic for the particle cores as a whole, the range of high q values for its local sub-structure, i.e. the crystallites.

We found that the shape of the scattering curves of the magnetic nanoparticles with the larger MPS amplitudes discriminates apparently better between two types of scattering entities than that of the particles with the lower MPS-performance. Quantitavely, the Guinier radii of the high performing tracers are larger by 20% only but the particle density within the clusters is about twice as high than in low performing tracers. Furthermore, there are slight but significant differences in the Porod approximation, i.e. fractal dimension of the clustered core particles.

Corresponding Author: N. Gehrke, nicole.gehrke@nanopet.de

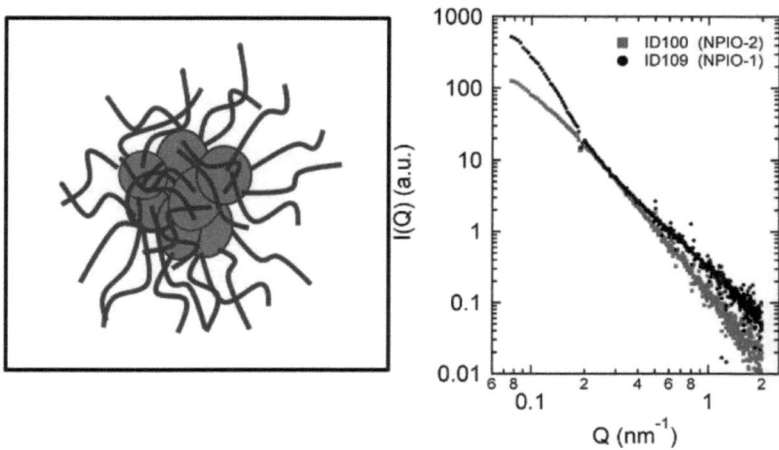

Fig.1: Schematic diagram of the multicore particle type investigated here and the X-ray scattering intensity I(Q) of two of those particles, NPIO-1 and NPIO-2, as a function of the magnitude of the scattering vector Q in double-logarithmic representation. The scattering data are corrected for signal background and smearing effects due to the slit collimation.

[1] Gehrke et al *"The Potential of Clustered Core Magnetic Particles for MPI"*, IEEE XPlore (2013), DOI 10.1109/IWMPI.2013.6528368

[2] B. Chu and T. Liu *"Characterization of nanoparticles by scattering techniques"* Journal of Nanoparticle Research (2000) 2: 29–41

Acknowledgements: This work was supported by the German Federal Ministry of Economics and Technology grant No. KF2725002UW2.

Corresponding Author: N. Gehrke, nicole.gehrke@nanopet.de

P47 PRODUCTION OF MONOSIZED MAGNETIC MICROSPHERES BY MICROFLUIDIC FLOW FOCUSING

Mehrdad Bokharaei[1], Silvio Dutz[2], Urs O. Häfeli[1]

[1]University of British Columbia, Faculty of Pharmaceutical Sciences, Vancouver, Canada
[2]Ilmenau University of Technology, Institute of Biomedical Engineering and Informatics, Germany

Biodegradable microspheres made from the polyesters poly(lactic acid) (PLA), poly(lactic-co-glycolic acid) (PLGA), and poly(caprolactone) (PCL) can be made with highly uniform size distribution with a method called flow focusing. In this method, the polymer is dissolved in chloroform and pumped through an orifice on a microfluidic glass chip. At the same time, a much higher (30x-100x) flow of an aqueous solution with a surface active agent (here polyvinyl alcohol) is pumped through the same orifice and "focuses" the stream of phase. Due to the pressure difference between inlet and the outlet of the orifice, the stream breaks up into monosized droplets. On the way out of the microfluidic chip, the solvent is extracted into the surrounding water phase, and single monosized microspheres form. We have earlier shown that this method works well, that it can produce microspheres of between 2.8 µm and 35 µm with a standard deviation of +/- 1.5 µm, and that we even can use it for the delivery of Tc-99m radiation to diagnose lung diseases. In the current work, we have now additionally made the microspheres magnetic by encapsulating appropriately coated magnetic nanoparticles into the polymeric bulk phase. Under controlled operational conditions, magnetic microspheres were produced with narrow size distribution (standard deviations of less than 5%) and a loading efficiency of magnetite up to 50% of the polymer dry weight. Such microspheres are promising for theranostics by combining magnetically guided targeting of the particles to their target location, imaging and localization of the particles by MPI or MRI, and drug release which can be triggered or enhanced by a local temperature increase realized by hyperthermia. In this presentation, details of the magnetic nanoparticle coatings necessary for the preparation of magnetic microspheres and their magnetic characterizations will be shown. Magnetic particle imaging spectra as well as hyperthermia data will be discussed.

Acknowledgments

This research was supported by a Canadian Institutes of Health Research (CIHR) and Natural Sciences and Engineering Research Council (NSERC) grant.

Corresponding Author: M. Bokharaei, mbokhara@interchange.ubc.ca

P48 VISCOSITY AFFECTED DETERMINATION OF IRON CONCENTRATION OF MPI TRACERS BASED ON MCT

Christina Debbeler, Kerstin Lüdtke-Buzug

Institute of Medical Engineering, University of Lübeck, Germany

The design and characterization of iron oxide tracer material suitable for Magnetic Particle Imaging (MPI) is a crucial part of the imaging chain. Considering the toxic effects of iron oxide tracers being injected overdosed, a thorough characterization of the ferrofluid regarding core diameter, volume, surface structure, and iron concentration using techniques such as Magnetic Particle Spectroscopy (MPS) or Photon Cross-correlation Spectroscopy (PCCS) is essential. A phantom has been constructed and an evaluation software has been implemented for micro Computed Tomography (µCT) based determination of the iron concentration of ferrofluids. This concept offers an alternative to photometry and atomic absorption spectroscopy. Measurements have been carried out with a Skyscan 1172 high-resolution µCT (Skyscan, Belgium) and reconstruction of the acquired data was realized with the Feldkamp, Davis and Kress approach (software: NRecon, Skyscan, Belgium).

In a first step, the scanning parameters for the µCT experiments had to be determined. Based on the results of a recent study [1], a tube voltage of 40 kV and an X-ray beam filtration with a 0.5 mm aluminum source filter has been chosen for iron concentration determination. Several measurements of ferrofluids with different concentrations were performed and statistically evaluated. Under the abovementioned conditions, it could be demonstrated that the measured mean attenuation value, represented as grey value in the µCT image, is proportional to the iron concentration. Using a linear calibration functional it is therefore possible to determine the concentration of any ferrofluid sample, based on a superparamagnetic iron oxide (SPIO) dispersion in the same solvent.

These first results indicate that a determination of the ferrofluid concentration using µCT is possible. Besides the tube voltage and the X-ray beam filtration, further parameters affect the accuracy of the measurements. This includes, for instance, the influence of the temperature on the density and in turn on the iron concentration of the fluid. Actually, the temperature of the sample may be increased, if several µCT scans are performed in a short time interval. Furthermore, a change of temperature influences the viscosity of the tracer suspension. Since liquid solutions have been used in all experiments, the influence of the viscosity on the CT attenuation value has to be evaluated as well.

In this contribution, µCT measurements of tracer material have been carried out under variation of temperature and viscosity. It can be demonstrated that the viscosity of the liquid matrix affects the concentration-attenuation calibration function. However, if the temperature-viscosity relation is known for the liquid matrix of the SPIO nanoparticles, µCT can be used for estimation of the iron concentration. This knowledge is a crucial step in characterizing tracer material and must be correlated with the results of further investigations using MPS and PCCS.

Acknowledgements:

The research leading to these results has received funding from the European Union Seventh Framework Programme (FP7/2007-2013) under grant agreement n°604448.

[1] C. Debbeler, J. Mueller, and K. Lüdtke-Buzug: Micro CT-based validation of iron concentration for MPI tracers, in: International Workshop on Magnetic Particle Imaging (IWMPI), 2013, IEEE Xplore, DOI: 10.1109/IWMPI.2013.6528337

Corresponding Author: C. Debbeler, debbeler@imt.uni-Lübeck.de

P49 DEVELOPMENT OF SUPERPARAMAGNETIC SURFACE COATINGS

Kerstin Lüdtke-Buzug, Christina Debbeler

Institute of Medical Engineering, University of Lübeck, Germany

Since it was first published in 2005, the greatest potential for Magnetic Particle Imaging (MPI) is seen in medical applications. However, dual-use applications of MPI, for instance, in safety engineering, quality assurance, and various other technical fields are interesting as well.

The development of superparamagnetic iron oxide nanoparticles (SPIONs) dispersed in polymers opens a wide field of potential applications. For instance, these polymers, such as polyethylene, polypropylene, and polyurethane, may be used for surface coatings of medical instruments. This is of particular interest, because superparamagnetic coatings of endoscopes or catheters would allow for MPI-guided minimally invasive surgical interventions. Additionally, structured SPION coatings may find applications as security labels or fraud-resistant badges in security-sensitive areas. Further, superparamagnetic nanoparticles may be combined with synthetic polymers, such as poly(tetrafluoroethylene) or polyethylene, for the production of surgical instruments.

In this contribution, experiments with metallic anti-rust protection coatings will be presented. It can be demonstrated that these materials show an acceptable, but poor magnetic response. However, when selecting particular magnetic coatings for surfaces of surgical instruments, special attention has to be paid to biocompatibility. Although the conventional anti-rust protection coatings gave an acceptable signal response in MPS, they cannot be used as coating of medical instruments due to their bio-incompatibility. In a second experiment, it is reported on coating results obtained with self-synthesized water-solved superparamagnetic iron oxide nanoparticles combined with different synthetic resin varnish. To obtain homogenous particle dispersion, nanoparticles have to be given in a fast process to the polymer and the mixture has to be homogenized by vigorous stirring. Consecutively, the homogenized mixture must be dried while applied to the surface materials, such as plastic layers or other tubing material.

The coating materials, metallic anti-rust protection coatings and the self-synthesized water-solved superparamagnetic iron oxide nanoparticles, have been analyzed with respect to their MPI responsiveness with magnetic particle spectroscopy (MPS). The materials have been analyzed in three different conditions, i.e. a) the pure particle suspension, b) particles fixed in a polymer, and c) the coated materials. In this comparison, the resulting harmonic decay plots of the MPS signal did not show any significant difference for the self-synthesized particles. However, it has been demonstrated that the magnetic response of surface coatings based on self-manufactured magnetic nanoparticles exceeds the magnetization response of metallic anti-rust surface protection coatings by far.

Corresponding Author: K. Lüdtke-Buzug, luedtke-buzug@imt.uni-Lübeck.de

P50 NOVEL DEVELOPED SUPERPARAMAGNETIC DEXTRAN COATED IRON OXIDE NANOPARTICLES (SPION) AS A POTENTIAL TOOL FOR HNSCC TUMOR CELL DETECTION AND ITS INFLUENCE ON THE BIOLOGICAL PROPERTIES

Ralph Pries[1], Antje Lindemann[1], Kerstin Lüdtke-Buzug[2], Barbara Wollenberg[1]

[1]Department of Otorhinolaryngology, University Hospital of Schleswig-Holstein, Campus Lübeck, Germany
[2]Institute of Medical Engineering, University of Lübeck, Germany

Purpose:
Research in biomedical engineering is still at the beginning to explore its possibilities. Although the imaging technology is already elementary for diagnostic and therapy in medical use, fundamental further developments are useful. A new revolutionary imaging technology is magnetic particle imaging (MPI). The development of a three-dimensional MPI scanner and a belonging superparamagnetic iron oxide nanoparticle (SPION) are in early stages. Here, we report the biocompatibility and biosafety of the dextran-coated MPI tracer of the University of Lübeck (UL-D) IMT.

Experimental Design:
We focused on UL-D induced impacts on the biological properties of head and neck squamous cell carcinoma (HNSCC) cells and their cellular uptake efficiency in comparison to the contrast agent Resovist, which is the gold standard for MPI.

Results:
UL-D and Resovist were taken up in vitro by human head and neck cancer cells, showed good labeling efficiencies and an accumulation. Flow cytometry analysis demonstrated a dose and time dependent, Resovist induced, apoptosis whereas the cell viability of UL-D labeled cells was not influenced. We observed decreased cell proliferation in response to increased SPION concentrations. The cellular migration and the intracellular production of reactive oxygen species (ROS) were not impaired. Tumor necrosis factor alpha (TNF-α) and the interleukins -6 (IL-6) -8 (IL-8) and -1 beta (IL-1ß) were measured indicating inflammatory responses. Only UT-SCC-60A, labeled with > 0.5 mM Resovist, showed a significant increase of IL-1ß expression.

Conclusions:
Our data suggest UL-D SPIONs as a promising tracer material for innovative tumor cell analyzes with the aid of MPI.

Corresponding Author: R. Pries, rallepries@yahoo.de

P51 — A SIZE-RESOLVED ANALYSIS OF ENCAPSULATED IRON OXIDE NANOPARTICLES AND RESOVIST®

Jan Niehaus[1], Sören Becker[2], Christian Schmidtke[2], Arthur Feld[2], Horst Weller[2]

[1]Center for Applied Nanotechnology (CAN GmbH), Hamburg, Germany
[2]University of Hamburg, Department of Physical Chemistry, Germany

Today superparamagnetic iron oxide nanoparticles (SPIOs) are used to form contrast agents with improved sensitivity and specificity. Their magnetic read-out in MRI or MPI measurements avoids risks which occur from ionizing (CT) or radioactive (PET) radiation. In difference to MRI the Magnetic Particle Imaging (MPI) measures the magnetic properties of iron oxide nanoparticles themselves and not their influence on the surrounding tissue. Therefore the properties of the used particles have an even larger influence on the resulting signal.

To yield a high quality contrast agent the used SPIOs should be monodispers with well defined and reproducible properties. This kind of particles can typically be produced by thermal decomposition reactions with diameters only between 5 and 20 nm. Also these particles are often dispersible in non polar solvents only, so a phase transfer after the synthesis is needed.

Nowadays mainly RESOVIST® is used in MPI studies as it yields stronger signals compared to the contrast agents based on above described monodisperse iron oxide particles. Unfortunately RESOVIST® is a rather divers system consisting of small crystalline particles as well as larger agglomerates of these (see TEM images shown in figure 1). It is known that only a small proportion of the whole sample actually contributes to the signal. Here we present the results of an investigation in which RESOVIST® was separated into different fraction using the asymmetric flow field-flow fractionation technique (AF4). MPS measurements of the different fractions are shown together with detailed TEM analysis.

In addition, we have continued to work on the reproducibility and up-scaling of our iron oxide nanoparticle synthesis. These particles can be used for our continuous flow phase transfer approach (CFPTA) described on the last meetings. Using this technique we can produce clustered iron oxide nanoparticles of different cluster sizes to tune their magnetic properties. To compare these results with RESOVIST® we have used AF4 to split these already well defined samples into several fractions with even narrower cluster size distribution. MPS measurements and HRTEM analysis will be shown.

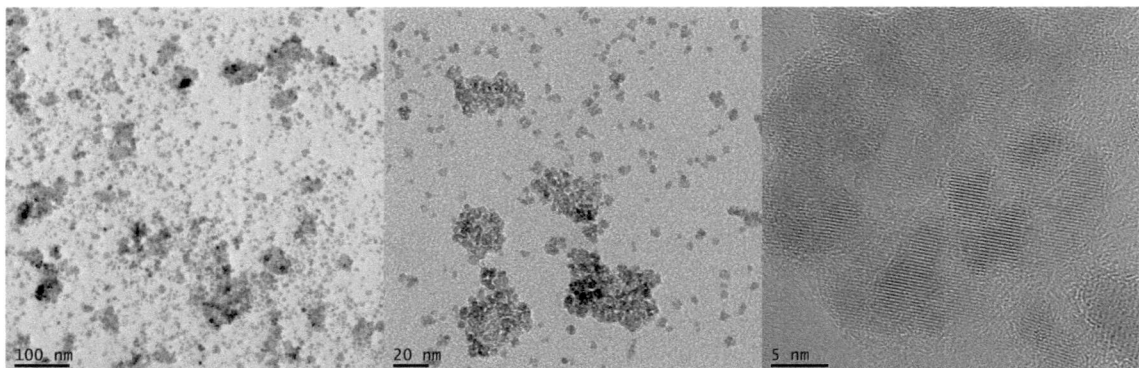

Figure 1: TEM images of RESOVIST®

Corresponding Author: J. Niehaus, niehaus@can-hamburg.de

P52 INFLUENCE ON MPI PROPERTIES OF MULTILAYER IRON OXIDE CORE

Hugo Groult[1,2], Nils Dennis Nothnagel[3], Jesus Ruiz-Cabello[1], Fernando Herranz[1]

[1]*Advanced imaging unit, CNIC (Spanish National Cardiovascular Research Centre), Madrid, Spain*
[2]*CIBER de Enfermedades Respiratorias, Mallorca, Spain*
[3]*Philips Healthcare Spain, Madrid, Spain*

Magnetic Particle Imaging (MPI) is a new imaging modality for preclinical and with a promising future in clinical investigation. The technique consists in detecting directly the spatial distribution of superparamagnetic iron oxide nanoparticles (SPIO) for high-resolution images. [1] This new medical imaging field opens many promising perspectives and it has opened extensive research for improving not only physics aspects of the system [2] but also SPIOs likely to display the best signal for MPI [3]. Indeed SPIOs have a major influence on the quality and sensitivity of the image, therefore developing suitable candidates for MPI is crucial for the future and the development of this technique [4]. It has been shown that higher magnetic moment is favourable for the resolution whereas long time of demagnetization is detrimental for the sensitivity [1]. As these two parameters are strongly but inversely linked with the diameter of the magnetite core, a fair balance has been reported to be around 30 nm core size. However until now the multiple influences of the SPIOs structure for optimal MPI signals remain fuzzy and the best performing and commonly used tracer is still the "old" Resovist.

In order to understand better how the magnetic moment and the size of the SPIOs affect the MPI image quality ; we prepared sets of three nanoparticles (NPs) which core diameter were increased by the addition of one and then two magnetite layers (ie. shell). The magnetic particle spectroscopy (MPS) signals of the three nanoparticles obtained (core-NPs, core@shell1-NPs, core@shell1@shell2-NPs) were measured and influence of the core size demonstrated. A nanoparticle prepared by a one-pot synthesis with a core of the same size than the core@shell1@shell2-NPs was used to consider as well the influence of the multiple layer structure. Indeed, the magnetization studies shown that the layer structure modified the magnetic properties. These data together with the MPS measurements were discussed. Moreover the results and influences were assesed and confirmed with 3 different sets of NP type : PEG (Mn=600) coated Fe_3O_4, oleic acid coated Fe_3O_4 and albumin coated Fe_3O_4.

[1] B. Gleich and J. Weizenecker, Tomographic imaging using the nonlinear response of magnetic particles, Nature, 435:7046, p. 1214–1217, 2005.

[2] Saritas, Emine U, Patrick W Goodwill, Laura R Croft, Justin J Konkle, Kuan Lu, Bo Zheng, and Steven M Conolly, Magnetic Particle Imaging (MPI) for NMR and MRI Researchers, Journal of Magnetic Resonance, 229, p. 116–126, 2013.

[3] Ferguson RM, Khandhar AP, Krishnan KM, Tracer design for magnetic particle imaging, J. Appl. Phys, 111(7), 2012.

Corresponding Author: H. Groult, hugo.groult@externo.cnic.es

P53 COMPARISON OF SOME MAGNETIC MULTICOMPONENT NANOPARTICLES FOR BIOMEDICAL APPLICATIONS

Nurcan Dogan[1], Ayhan Bingölbali[2], M. Asilturk[3], Z. Yeşil[4]

[1] Science Faculty-Department of Physics, Gebze Institute of Technology, Turkey
[2] Yildiz Technical University, Department of Bioengineering, Esenler-Istanbul, Turkey
[3] Akdeniz University, Department of Metallurgy Engineering, Antalya, Turkey
[4] Akdeniz University, Department of Chemistry, Antalya, Turkey

Magnetic nanoparticles (NPs) are increasingly important in many biomedical applications, such as drug delivery, hyperthermia, and magnetic resonance imaging (MRI) contrast enhancement. To build the most effective magnetic nanoparticle systems for various biomedical applications, characteristics of particle, including size, surface chemistry, magnetic properties, and toxicity have to be fully investigated. In this work, effects of some production methods of the magnetic nanoparticles for the bio-medical applications are discussed. In this investigation, multicomponent ferrite nanoparticles were prepared by the hydrothermal synthesis, sol-gel, and solid state methods. In addition, x-ray powder diffractometry (XRD), scanning electron microscopy (SEM), and vibrating scanning magnetometer (VSM) were used to characterize the structural, morphological and magnetic properties of the nanoparticles. The size and crystal structure of the nanoparticles were characterized by using XRD results. The magnetic properties of the samples were performed for each sample at +/-80 kOe by Quantum Design Physical Properties System (PPMS). The temperature dependence of field cooled (FC) magnetization of the samples have been compared in this work.

Corresponding Author: N. Dogan, nurcandogan80@gmail.com

P54 MEASURING DIPOLAR INTERACTIONS AND MAGNETIC CORRELATIONS IN SELF-ASSEMBLED NANOPARTICLE SUPERSTRUCTURES WITH ELECTRON HOLOGRAPHY

Marco Beleggia[1], Miriam Varon[2], Tekeshi Kasama[1], Richard J Harrison[3], Rafal E Dunin-Borkowski[4], Victor F Puntes[2], Cathrine Frandsen[5]

[1]Center for Electron Nanoscopy, Technical University of Denmark, Lyngby, Denmark
[2]Institut Catala' de Nanotecnologia, Campus U A B, Barcelona, Spain
[3]Department of Earth Sciences, University of Cambridge, United Kingdom
[4]Ernst Ruska Centre for Microscopy and Spectroscopy with Electrons and Peter Gruenberg Institute, Research Centre Juelich, Germany
[5]Department of Physics, Technical University of Denmark, Lyngby, Denmark

Assemblies (or superstructures) of magnetic nanoparticles are a novel class of magnetic materials, often represented by a superlattice of particles. In such materials, inter-particle exchange interactions may be negligible, while dipolar interactions dominate. As a result, magnetic superstructures behave differently from conventional magnets and their properties may be controlled and tuned by selecting the spacing and compositions of the constituents. We have studied dipolar interactions in self-assembled Cobalt nanoparticle elongated superstructures using off-axis electron holography in the transmission electron microscope. The technique enables the orientation and magnitude of the magnetic moment of each nanoparticle in an array to be determined and correlated with the structural properties of the superlattice, including the degree of structural order and their size distribution. Our study reveals that dipolar interactions are sufficiently strong to support long-range ferromagnetic order, even when the superlattice of nanoparticles is highly disordered. This observation supports the possibility of creating amorphous dipolar magnets, in contrast to the expectation that a disordered dipolar system is likely to lead to spin-glass behavior. Chain-like assemblies of 15 nm e-Co particles were prepared with an oleic acid coating on a carbon substrate (with no external magnetic field applied). For chains that are wider than 1 particle across, the particles are typically assembled into triangular (close-packed) lattices, although square lattice arrangements are also occasionally seen. We used off-axis electron holography to map the projected magnetic fields of several elongated nanoparticle assemblies non-invasively with a nominal spatial resolution of 6.3 nm. The data set was acquired at remanence after applying an off-plane field of 2 T to the specimen, and reveals the magnetic moment topography of each chain directly. In order to quantify dipolar ferromagnetic order, we estimated the magnitude and orientation of the magnetic moment of each individual particle from electron holography data, in particular by measuring the two components of the shape-corrected phase gradient, a quantity that turns out to be proportional to the local density of magnetic moments (magnetization). The measurements were correlated with the geometrical arrangements of the particles. For each pair of particles, we measured the spatial separation between their centers and the angular difference between their moments, from which magnetic and lattice order parameters were determined. Our results show that short-range magnetic order with small domains dominates the initial states, with the local magnetic order (ferromagnetic or antiferromagnetic) often depending on the particle lattice (triangular or square, respectively). In contrast, at remanence after saturation, overall dipolar ferromagnetic order persists even in case of a non-triangular lattice. We interpret our results as supporting the existence of amorphous dipolar ferromagnets: i.e., dipolar ferromagnetism in elongated nanoparticle assemblies even in the absence of underlying crystallinity. Our results also demonstrate that electron holography is a technique capable of capturing the nanoscale magnetic fields generated by magnetized particles, and of providing quantitative information on their magnetic moment as well as on their response to an applied external field.

Corresponding Author: M. Beleggia, marco.beleggia@cen.dtu.dk

Poster

Medical Applications

P55 SPIO DETECTION AND DISTRIBUTION IN BIOLOGICAL TISSUE - A MURINE MPI-SNLB BREAST CANCER MODEL

Dominique Finas[1], Kristin Baumann[2], Lotta Sydow[2], Katja Heinrich[2], Achim Rody[2], Ksenija Gräfe[3], Kerstin Lüdtke-Buzug[3], Thorsten Buzug[3]

[1] Department of Obstetrics and Gynecology, Evangelic Hospital Bielefeld, Germany and University of Lübeck, Germany
[2] Department of Obstetrics and Gynecology, University of Lübeck, Germany
[3] Institute of Medical Engineering, University of Lübeck, Germany

Surgical breast cancer related staging with radical axillary lymph node extraction was mandatory in past times. High morbidity and significant loss of QoL was inevitable. By introduction of the concept of sentinel lymph node biopsy (SNLB), these adverse effects decreased. Detection of SNLs is realized by the use of dyes and radio nuclides as tracer substances. These tracers can be replaced by super paramagnetic iron oxide nano particles (SPIOs) in the near future. Magnetic particle imaging (MPI) guided 3D-real time-imaging and a distinct localization of SPIOs can be achieved in SNLB by the use of magnetic particle imaging (MPI). However, qualitative and quantitative enrichment of SPIOs in biologic tissue particularly the axillary lymphatic tissue is unexplored until now. We aim to prove the principle of SNLB with MPI within a healthy and than in a tumor bearing mouse model with metastatic axillary lymph nodes in breast cancer. Axillary tissue, surrounding tissues and tissue from the whole body are analyzed with the following techniques: histology, Prussian blue staining, electron microscopy, atomic absorption spectrometry and MPI spectrometry. We found that the SPIOs moves from the injection site through the lymph-fat tissue to the axillary region and finally into the axillary lymph nodes. SPIOs follow traces of lymphatic vessels, respecting borders and spaces between different tissues. They accumulates near collagen fibers and distinct regions. We present our results of the approach of SNLB with MPI. Application of SPIOs and tracer detection in SNLs with MPI as a new SNLB technology are less complex and incriminating for patient and staff and makes SNLB more accurate. To realize this approach, a MPI hand probe for intra operative use is under construction. This simplifies SNL detection and helps to reduce axillary exploration morbidity by avoidance of intensive surgical quest. The tracer for MPI is easy to obtain and this makes the method accessible to all patients. The concept of SNLB by MPI can be applied in principle in all solid tumors.

Acknowledgments
This project is supported by the German Federal Ministry of Education and Research (BMBF Grant number 01EZ0912). It is also part of the University Research Program "Imaging of Disease Processes", University of Lübeck.

Corresponding Author: D. Finas, finas.d@arcor.de

P56 MAGNETIC IRON NANOPARTICLES AS USEFUL TOOL FOR DIRECTING AND DETECTING CELLS IN REGENERATIVE MEDICINE

Marc Schwarz[1], **Philipp Tripal**[1], Stefan Lyer[1], Frank Wiekhorst[2], Tobias Engelhorn[3], Tobias Struffert[3], Arnd Doerfler[3], Lutz Trahms[2], Christoph Alexiou[1]

[1]ENT-Department; Section for Experimental Oncology and Nanomedicine and Department of Neuroradiology, University Hospital Erlangen, Germany
[2]Physikalisch-Technische Bundesanstalt, Berlin, Germany
[3]Department of Neuroradiology, University Hospital of Erlangen, Germany

In regenerative medicine until now mostly tissue-engineered skin is on focus for replacement of damaged tissue in patients. If it comes down to more complex organs or endothelialized vessel grafts, however, there still exist several unsolved problems. Therefore it still remains a challenge to produce organs that consist of more than one cell type in different layers, since it is not yet possible to direct cells to their dedicated position on or in a matrix. On the other hand it is difficult to view the positioning of the cells in complex matrices. These problems could possibly be solved by loading cells with magnetic nanoparticles and the use of magnetic fields to maneuver those cells to their dedicated position. The successful positioning can then be monitored by techniques that are able to image magnetic or quantify nanoparticles (e.g. magnetic resonance imaging or magnetic particle imaging).

As a first proof of principle we chose to seed endothelial cells three-dimensionally onto the inner wall of a cell culture tube as first model for an endothelialized vessel graft.

Therefore we cultivated Huvec cells under standard conditions and added different concentrations of Resovist as standard magnetic nanoparticles and magnetic nanoparticles developed in our own lab (SEON-TE). After 24h the cells were harvested and transferred into a cell culture tube. A radial symmetric magnetic field was used to pull the cells to the wall of the tube. Medium was removed 24 hours, 72 hours or 96 hours after the cells adhered to the tube and the cells were fixed. To visualize iron within the cells we used Prussian blue staining and 3T MRI (TRIO, Siemens, Germany) equipped with an 11cm loop coil (Siemens, Germany) using T_1-, T_2- and SWI sequences. To quantify the iron amount within the cells we employed Magnetic Particle Spectroscopy. We obtained a construct that consisted of one or more cell layers and could visualize iron in all samples using Prussian blue staining and MRI, which was also capable of imaging the loaded cells.

Acknowledgements:
The authors would like to thank the Else Kroener-Fresenius Stiftung and the DFG (SPP 1681, AL552/5-1, TR408/5-2).

Corresponding Author: M. Schwarz, Marc.Schwarz@uk-erlangen.de;
P. Tripal, Philipp.Tripal@uk-erlangen.de

P57 USE OF RED BLOOD CELLS TO PROLONG THE IN VIVO LIFE SPAN OF IRON-BASED CONTRAST AGENTS FOR MRI AND MPI

Mauro Magnani[1,2], Antonella Antonelli[1], Carla Sfara[1], Jürgen Rahmer[3], Bernhard Gleich[3], Jörn Borgert[3]

[1]Department of Biomolecular Sciences, University of Urbino "Carlo Bo", Italy
[2]EryDel S.p.A., Urbino, Italy
[3]Philips Technologie GmbH Innovative Technologies, Research Laboratories, Hamburg, Germany

In the field of nanotechnology, superparamagnetic iron oxide (SPIO) and ultra small superparamagnetic iron oxide (USPIO) nanoparticles have been developed as magnetic resonance imaging (MRI) contrast agents. To date, there are clinically approved contrast agents for MRI that would also be suitable for Magnetic Particle Imaging (MPI). It has further been found that the MPI signal is mainly generated by particles with a 30 nm magnetic core diameter [1]. The MPI applications can be realized by imaging a bolus of iron-oxide nanoparticles injected into the blood stream. Resovist®, a commercial SPIO-based MRI liver contrast agent, has been successfully used as an in vivo MPI tracer for real-time visualization of the bolus passage through the heart of a mouse [2]. However, these SPIO nanoparticles are most quickly removed from the blood stream by the mononuclear phagocyte system which limits the applicability of such compounds in MPI. The use of longer blood half-time tracer materials would make MPI highly suitable for e.g. perfusion imaging and/or continuous monitoring. In this contest, we have proposed a method of SPIO nanoparticles encapsulation into red blood cells (RBCs) that avoids their fast uptake by the reticuloendothelial system, increasing the blood circulation half-life of nanoparticles [3]. The magnetic characterization of SPIO-loaded RBCs and their potential as tracer material for MPI has been demonstrated [4]. Resovist® has been chosen for its good MPI performance and the fact that its suitability for RBCs entrapment has already been established. Despite the reduced sensitivity and resolution resulting from the size selection effect, and despite the difficulties related to the application of the loading procedure to mice instead of humans, the sensitivity of the experimental MPI instrumentation allows dynamic imaging up to several hours after Resovist®-loaded RBC injection. By loading RBCs with Resovist®, MPI of the blood pool of living mice is feasible several hours after injection with current MPI equipment. This has been demonstrated by visualization of cardiac motion in MPI and by determination of the concentration of iron loaded RBCs in the blood using MPS. These results prove the efficacy of the RBCs loading method for increasing the blood retention time of iron oxide nanoparticles. Current and future improvements in particle performance, loading procedure, MPI hardware and calibration as well as the transfer to human anatomy are expected to increase the signal levels and thus improve image quality strongly. Therefore, one of the challenges is to find new synthesis protocols and optimize next generation nanoparticle tracer materials. Recently, we performed studies on the encapsulation into human and murine RBCs of a new contrast agent, the P904 provided by Guerbet, an USPIO nanoparticle suspension. The results have shown an efficient entrapment into RBCs and an high stability of P904-loaded RBCs in the mice vascular system respect to free P904 suspension.

New MPI-optimized particles may be used for the RBC loading procedure. The circulation survival of new optimal RBC-encapsulated MPI tracers will be evaluated with the aim to use these new biomimetic contructs in biomedical applications such as angiography and perfusion imaging.

[1] Weizenecker J, Borgert J, Gleich B. A simulation study on the resolution and sensitivity of magnetic particle imaging. Phys Med Biol. 2007; 52(21): 6363-74.

[2] Weizenecker J, Gleich B, Rahmer J, Dahnke H & Borgert J. Three-dimensional real-time in vivo magnetic particle imaging. Phys Med Biol. 2009; 54(5): L1-L10.

Corresponding Author: M. Magnani, Mauro.magnani@uniurb.it

[3] Antonelli A, Sfara C, Battistelli S, Canonico B, et al. New strategies to prolong the in vivo life span of iron-based contrast agents for MRI. PLOS ONE 2013; 8 (10): e78542.

[4] Rahmer J, Antonelli A, Sfara C, Tiemann B, Gleich B, Magnani M, Weizenecker J and Borgert J. Nano-particle encapsulation in red blood cells enables blood pool magnetic particle imaging hours after injection. Phys Med Biol. 2013; 58 (12): 3965-3977.

Corresponding Author: M. Magnani, Mauro.magnani@uniurb.it

P58 TIME BEHAVIOR OF FERROFLUIDS UNDER LIQUID STREAM CONDITIONS IN MAGNETIC DRUG TARGETING APPLICATIONS: SIMULATION AND EXPERIMENTAL INVESTIGATION

I. Slabu[1,2], A. Röth[3], G. Guentherodt[2], T. Schmitz-Rode[1], M. Baumann[1]

[1]Applied Medical Engineering, Medical Faculty, Helmholtz Institute, RWTH Aachen University, Germany
[2]Physics Institute, RWTH Aachen University, Germany
[3]Department of General, Visceral and Transplantation Surgery, University Hospital Aachen, Germany

The interaction of magnetic fields with single suspended superparamagnetic iron oxides (SPIO) in blood flow is described in a new magnetic targeting simulation model. Based on FEM simulations this model traces the SPIO in a vessel and counts the number of SPIO that are adsorbed at the vessel wall facilitating a quantification of the efficiency of the targeting system. It has been constructed for endoluminal tumors (e. g. pancreatic ductal adenocarcinoma, esophagus adenocarcinoma or bile duct Klatskin tumors) which permit the minimally invasive endoscopic insertion of permanent magnets very close to the tumor site where a strong magnetic field and a high magnetic field gradient are achieved. The simulation model was applied to the respective physical and chemical properties of SPIO, the blood flow properties and different magnetic field configurations generated by permanent magnets. For instance, an iron adsorption of 5.5×10^{-4} mg to the vessel wall within one hour was calculated for a permanent magnet with a magnetic field strength of 0.3 T and a gradient of 400 T/m, a blood flow velocity of 0.03 cm/s and a SPIO mass fraction of 3.125×10^{-4}.

The simulation model was tested in a simple experimental set-up of an acrylic glass flow chamber modeling a vessel (see Figure 1). The experiments were performed with water (instead of blood) and 0.15 ml ferrofluid (colloidal SPIO), which was injected into the flow chamber and collected at the target site where a magnetic field was generated by a permanent magnet. The flow type was laminar and its velocity in the order of 1 cm/s. The time evolution of the ferrofluid accumulation was measured.

For this matter, an optical method of observation using a video camera was developed and showed that the accumulation of the ferrofluid takes place in four different phases. The first phase is a passage phase, in which the ferrofluid passes the target site without significantly being collected, followed by an accumulation phase which is characterized by an increase of the ferrofluid quantity at the chamber wall.

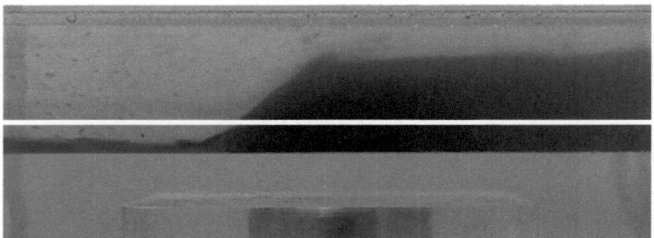

Figure 1: Side view of the flow chamber experiment. This screenshot was taken during the accumulation phase, see text.

In the third phase, parts of the ferrofluid are ashed away, and finally a stable accumulation is reached in phase four. Comparing the simulation and experimental results, it can be deduced that the calculated behavior corresponds well to the accumulation and saturation phases (second and fourth phases). The retarded start of accumulation (first phase) and the partial wash-away (third phase) could not yet be reproduced in the simulation model.

Corresponding Author: I. Slabu, slabu@hia.rwth-aachen.de

P59   TOWARD LOCALIZED IN VIVO BIOMARKER CONCENTRATION MEASUREMENTS

John B. Weaver[1], Daniel Reeves[2], Yipeng Shi[2], Alexander Hartov[3], Barjor Gimi[1], Krishnamurthy V. Nemani[1]

[1]*Department of Radiology, Dartmouth-Hitchcock Medical Center and Dartmouth College, One Medical Center Drive, Lebanon, US*
[2]*Department of Physics, Dartmouth College, Hanover, US*
[3]*Thayer School of Engineering, Dartmouth College, Hanover, US*

Magnetic spectroscopy of magnetic nanoparticles has been used to quantify the concentration of biomarker molecules in vitro. Spectroscopic methods were used to estimate the number of nanoparticles that are bound together by the targeted biomarker or signaling molecule [1]. The spectroscopic method has been termed magnetic spectroscopy of Brownian motion or MSB. To translate the technology to *in vivo* use: 1) The nanoparticles must be enclosed in porous shells [2] to keep the immune system from absorbing the nanoparticles and to maintain their physical location. 2) The chemistry must function in "dirty" environments where there are a wide variety of other molecules present. 3) The sensitivity must be improved to measure signaling molecules that are present in tissue in very low concentrations. We encapsulated targeted nanoparticles in porous alginate shells. The encapsulated nanoparticles were used to measure the concentration of single strand DNA in blood [1] demonstrating the ability to use the system in "dirty" environments using chemistry very similar to that used in ELISA [3]. The sensitivity was only a factor of four less than that in pure water. Finally, we demonstrate preliminary results from our efforts to increase the sensitivity of the spectroscopic system. We reduced the vibrational noise by gluing the windings of both the drive and pickup coils. We have explored two methods of reducing the feed-through signal induced in the pickup coils by the drive field: using a bridge to null the voltage from the pickup coil before the sample is placed and perpendicular field pickup coil actuated by a small static field. The resulting sensitivity for both methods was improved by three orders of magnitude. Further gains in sensitivity can be made by using lower noise electronics, magnetic shielding, increasing the affinity of the targeting and increasing the number of targeting molecules on each nanoparticle. The methods used to improve the sensitivity can be used on an existing mouse coil. The key elements of an *in vivo* system have been successfully demonstrated.

Corresponding Author: J. B. Weaver, john.b.weaver@dartmouth.edu

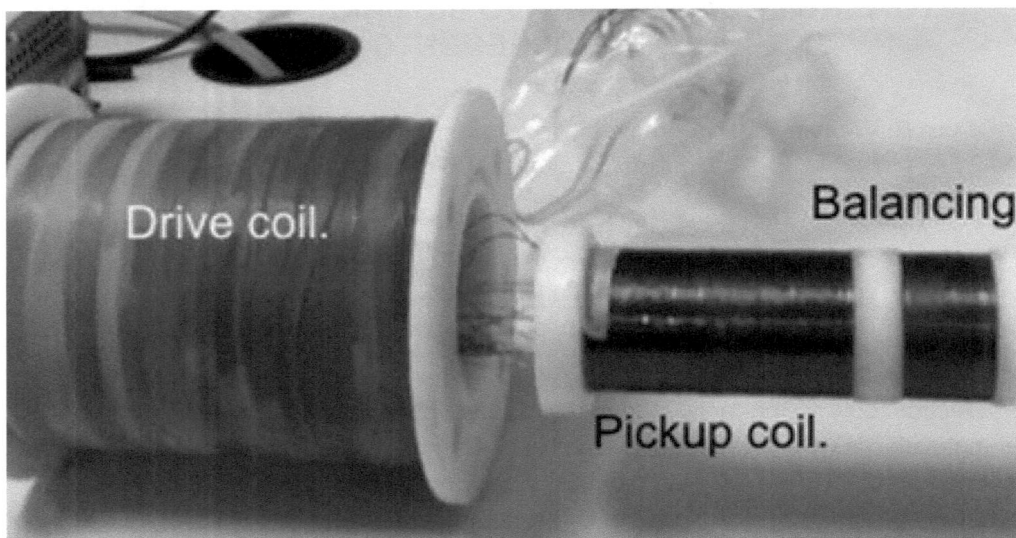

Figure 1: A prototype mouse coil for spectroscopic MSB measurements. The plastic parts were fabricated using 3D printing technology.

[1] X. Zhang, D.B. Reeves, I.M. Perreard, W.C. Kett, K.E. Griswold, B. Gimi, J.B. Weaver, Molecular sensing with magnetic nanoparticles using magnetic spectroscopy of nanoparticle Brownian motion, Biosensors and Bioelectronics, 50 (2013) 441-446.

[2] B. Gimi, J. Kwon, L. Liu, Y. Su, K. Nemani, K. Trivedi, Y. Cui, B. Vachha, R. Mason, W. Hu, J.B. Lee, Cell encapsulation and oxygenation in nanoporous microcontainers, Biomedical microdevices, 11 (2009) 1205-1212.

[3] E. Engvall;, P. Perlmann, Enzyme-Linked Immunosorbent Assay, Elisa, Journal of Immunology, 109 (1972) 129-135.

Corresponding Author: J. B. Weaver, john.b.weaver@dartmouth.edu

P60 FDTD ANALYSIS OF ELECTROMAGNETICALLY INDUCED HEATING AND BIO-HEAT TRANSFER FOR MAGNETIC FLUID HYPERTHERMIA

Wu Lei[1], Cheng Jingjing[2], Liu Wenzhong[2]

[1]School of Chemical Engineering and Environment, Beijing Institute of Technology, China
[2]School of Automation, Huazhong University of Science and Technology, Wuhan, China

In the report, we study the computational modeling of electromagnetically induced heating in Magnetic Fluid Hyperthermia. Due to the Brownian rotation and Neel relaxation of induced magnetic moments, ferrofluid can generate heat when exposed to an AC magnetic field. In order to destroy all tumors cells while prevent deleterious physiological responses, the input parameters such as the frequency and intensity of magnetic fields and complex susceptibility of ferrofluid should be determined precisely above all. In this study, the solution of Maxwell equation in a model of tumor and its neighboring tissues is coupled as input to the Penne's bio-heat equation. Both sets of equations are solved using the Finite Difference Time Domain (FDTD) method with Perfectly Matched Layers for absorbing boundary conditions. In this paper, we use a bilayered spherical model with blood perfusion and metabolism to simulate both the SAR patterns and temperature distribution in tumor region during hyperthermia therapy. And then a 2.0kW radio-frequency generator with 100 kHz-2MHz frequency range is developed to drive a custom-made multi-turns water-cooled coil, which generates a sufficient magnetic field inside it. Derived from the electromagnetic field simulation, the power density serves as input to the bio-heat transfer equation and therefore the heating generated by the ferrofluid is determined. The obtained results indicate that tumor region is heated without adversely affecting too much of the healthy region. Different boundary conditions and different blood perfusion rates have been taken into consideration in this paper.

[1] Lv, Y.-G., Z.-S. Deng, and J. Liu, "3-D numerical study on induced heating effects of embedded micro/nanoparticles on human body subject to external medical electromagnetic field," *IEEE Transactions on Nanobioscience*, Vol. 14, No.4, 284-292, 2005.

[2] Ch. Zhang, D.T. Johnson, Ch. S. Brazel, "Numerical study of the multiregion bio-heat equation to model magnetic fluid hyperthermia (MFH) using low Curie temperature nanoparticles," *IEEE Transactions on Nanobioscience*, Vol. 7, No.4, 267-275, 2008.

[3] J. Carrey, B. Mehdaoui and M. Respaud, "Simple models for dynamic hysteresis loop calculations of magnetic single-domain nanoparticles: Application to magnetic hyperthermia optimization", *J. Appl. Phys.*, Vol. 109, 083921-1 -083921-17, 2011

[4] D. Dołęga, and J. Barglik, "Computer modeling and simulation of radiofrequency thermal ablation," *Proceedings of International Conference on Electromagnetic Field, Health and Environment*, Coimbra, Portugal, May 2011.

Corresponding Author: W. Lei, wulei1121@gmail.com

P61 VISUALIZATION OF MAGNETIC NANOPARTICLES IN THE TUMOUR AREA AFTER INTRA-ARTERIAL OR INTRA-TUMOURAL APPLICATION

Stefan Lyer[1], **Marc Schwarz**[1,2], Tobias Engelhorn[2], Tobias Struffert[2], Arnd Dörfler[2], Christoph Alexiou[1]

[1]ENT-Department; Section for Experimental Oncology and Nanomedicine, University Hospital Erlangen, Germany
[2]Department of Neuroradiology, University Hospital Erlangen, Germany

Although some progress has been achieved in cancer treatment during the past decades this illness is still one of the leading causes of death, worldwide. The aim of new approaches nowadays is a personalized and target directed treatment of tumours, which should lead to more efficient therapies with an elongation of life accompanied by better quality of life. Here, the use of magnetic nanoparticles (SPIONs) is promising different options for cancer treatment as well as in situ treatment monitoring during therapy.

SPIONs can be used for drug delivery, like it is done in Magnetic Drug Targeting (MDT). It could be shown recently, that this approach can lead efficiently to complete tumour remissions after only one intaarterial application of Mitoxantrone loaded SPIONs. On the other hand SPIONS can be used for magnetically induced Hyperthermia of tumour tissue with alternating magnetic fields. Here intratumoural application of nanoparticles is the usual mode of application.

It is known already, that SPIONs can be used as imaging agents for MPI and MRI. In conventional MRI-scanners magnetic nanoparticles are causing either positive signals or signal extinction, dependent on their magnetic properties.

The aim of this initial study was to investigate *in vivo* the different distribution patterns of iron oxide nanoparticles in the region of a tumour after intraarterial or intratumoural application using a conventional clinical MRI-Scanner (Magneton TIM Trio, Siemens Healthcare, Erlangen, Germany). Therefore four New Zealand White Rabbits were implanted with kryokonserved VX2 tumour tissue at the left hind limb, subcutaneously. After the tumours had grown, MR-imaging was done before SPION-application, serving as control at day 0. Here, T_1-, T_2- and contrast enhanced T_1-sequenzes were used. On the next day the nanoparticles were applied either intraarterial through the *arteria femoralis* at the medial thigh with Magnetic Drug Targeting or by intratumoural injection. On day three, 24h after treatment, MR-imaging was done again using the same sequences. The images showed clearly different distribution patterns between the different application modes. Intraarterial administration right next to the tumour bulk under X-ray control lead to more "scattered" distributions and particles in the surrounding tissue of the tumours. The pattern of SPIONS injected directly showed very high and dense signals directly surrounding the area of injection, while no particles could be detected in the surrounding tissue.

In this preliminary study we could show, that it is possible to visualize *in vivo* the different biodistribution of SPION in a tumour after i.a. or i.t. administration. The most obvious differences were higher concentrations of nanoparticles after direct injection. On the other hand after i.a. MDT the nanoparticles could be found mostly in the vital area of the tumours and the surrounding tissue.)

In further studies MRI-sequences more susceptible for iron oxide signals or the use of Magnetic Particle Imaging could give even better results and more insight into the *in vivo* distribution of iron oxide nanoparticles for cancer treatment. In consequence this will lead to an efficient monitoring of the treatment of tumours by the use of magnetic iron oxide nanoparticles.

The authors would like to thank the Else Kroener-Fresenius Stiftung, the DFG (PAK 151, AL552/3-3) and the German Federal Ministery of Education and Research (BMBF) (*FKZ 13EX1012B*).

Corresponding Authors: S. Lyer, stefan.lyer@uk-erlangen.de;
M. Schwarz, marc.schwarz@uk-erlangen.de

P62 OPTIMIZATION OF ONCOLYTIC VIRUS/MAGNETIC-NANOPARTICLE-COMPLEXES FOR TUMOR THERAPY

Florian Wille[1], Olga Mykhaylyk[2], Jennifer Altomonte[3], Juliane Dworniczak[1], Isabella Almstätter[1], Ernst Rummeny[1], Oliver Ebert[3], Christian Plank[2], Rickmer Braren[1]

[1] Institut fuer diagnostische und interventionelle Radiologie, TU Muenchen, Germany
[2] Institut fuer experimentelle Onkologie und Therapieforschung, TU Muenchen, Germany
[3] 2. Medizinische Klinik und Poliklinik, TU Muenchen, Germany

Systemic application of oncolytic viruses for cancer therapy is greatly limited by the relative inefficiency of viral vectors to reach and infect their tumor targets, due to inactivation by blood components and sequestration by liver and spleen [1]. One approach to overcome this hurdle is to couple the virus with iron nanoparticles, which can then be targeted to the tumor using a magnet [2, 3]; however, the resulting complexes have a short plasma half-life and are susceptible to aggregation and emboli formation in vivo, which poses a major safety concern. **Aim**: Assembling of vesicular stomatitis virus (VSV) - Magnetic nanoparticle (MNP) complexes in combination with different shielding polymers for improvement of plasma half-life and a reduction of aggregation. **Methods**: Complexation of VSV and core-shell-type iron oxide MNPs, followed by shielding with different polymers (hyaluronic acid, poly-alpha-glutamic acid, poly-galacturonic acid, P6YE5C) using layer-by-layer self-assembling technique. Examination of hydrodynamic diameter, zeta-potential, magnetophoretic mobility and infectivity. Examination of blood-half-life in buffalo rats. **Results**: Complexation of VSV led to charge neutralization at a MNP-to-virus ratio of 19,5 fgFe/pfu. Complexes formulated at a ratio of 300fgFe/pfu showed a hydrodynamic diameter of 2016,67 (SD 399,85) and a zeta potential of 15,10 mV (SD 0,50). They were most effective in binding VSV with > 99% of the originally added virus bound as determined by magnetic sedimentation assay. Decoration with shielding polymers led to no relevant change of complex size, but to charge reversal; e.g. hyaluronic acid effectively changed the zeta potential from 14,2 mV (SD 0,33) to -20,18 mV (SD 0,61) at a polymer-to-iron (w/w) ratio of 10. In vitro infectivity and replication were not impaired. Preliminary in vivo experiments demonstrated a longer blood-half-life time of the shielded complexes and reduced toxicity. **Conclusion**: The use of shielding polymers leads to charge optimization of the VSV-MNP complexes without loss of oncolytic activity, indicating that this is a viable approach for improving the delivery and safety of magnetic-targeted oncolytic VSV therapy for cancer. Future studies aim at further characterization and the in vivo application of optimized complexes. **Keywords**: HCC, iron-oxide magnetic nanoparticle, Vesicular Stomatitis Virus, magnetic targeting

[1] Russell, S.J., K.W. Peng, and J.C. Bell, *Oncolytic virotherapy.* Nat Biotechnol, 2012. 30(7): p. 658-70.

[2] Zhang, Y., et al., Targeted delivery of human VEGF gene via complexes of magnetic nanoparticle-adenoviral vectors enhanced cardiac regeneration. PLoS One, 2012. 7(7): p. e39490.

[3] Anton, M., et al., Optimizing adenoviral transduction of endothelial cells under flow conditions. Pharm Res, 2012. 29(5): p. 1219-31.

Corresponding Author: F. Wille, florian.wille@mytum.de

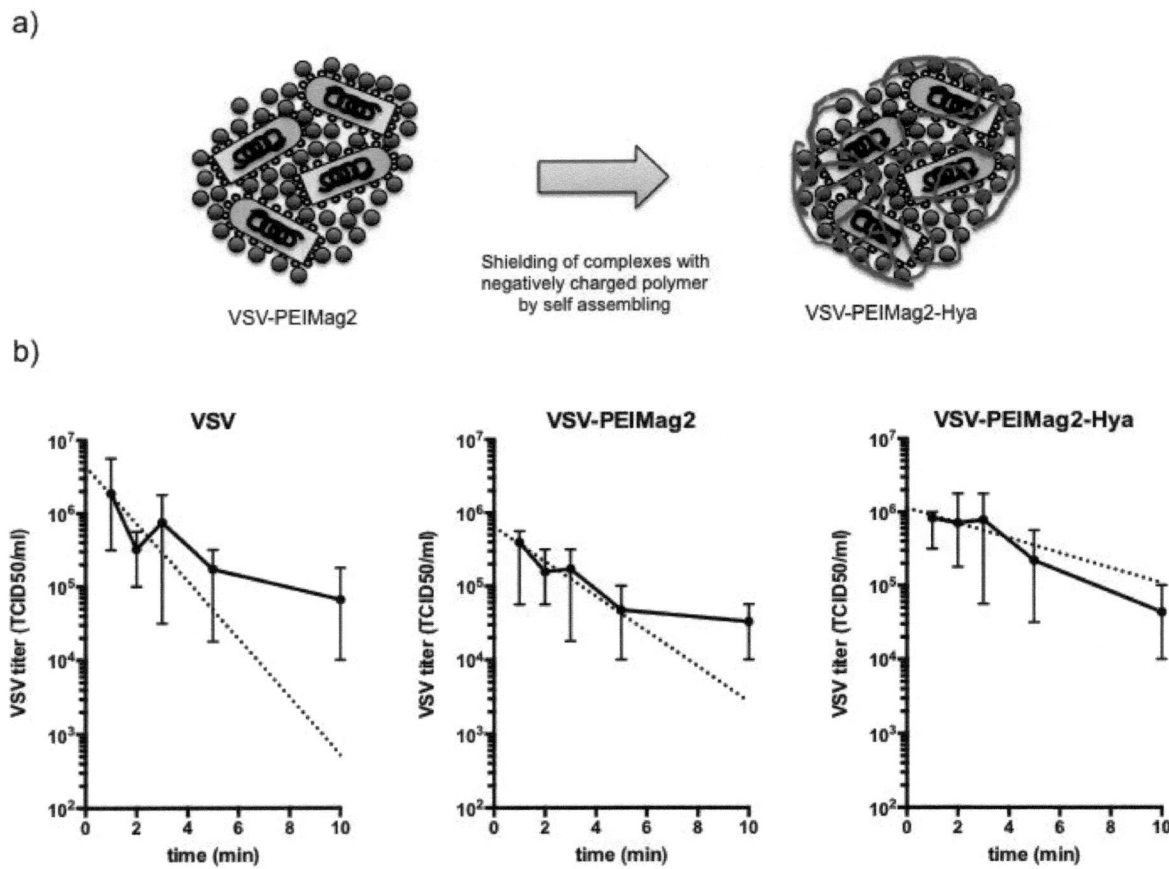

Figure: a) Schematic view of VSV-MNP complexes before (VSV-PEIMag2) and after shielding with hyaluronic acid (VSV-PEIMag2-Hya) b) Full-blood VSV titer in Buffalo rats after injection of 10^7pfu of VSV, VSV-PEIMag2 or VSV-PEIMag2-Hya, measured at 1,2,3,5 and 10 minutes after injection. The dotted lines show the exponential decay fitting curves. n=4 for the VSV and VSV-PEIMag2-Hya and n=3 for the VSV-PEIMag2 group. The error bars show the results range.

Corresponding Author: F. Wille, florian.wille@mytum.de

P63 MR IMAGING OF A SPIO-LABELED PATHOGEN IN VIVO: DISTRIBUTION OF PARASITIC PROTOZOAN ENTAMOEBA HISTOLYTICA IN THE LIVER OF A MOUSE MODEL AT 7T

Harald Ittrich[1], Thomas Ernst[1], Hannah Bernin[2], Gerhard Adam[1], Hannelore Lotter[2]

[1]*Department of Diagnostic and Interventional Radiology, University Medical Center Hamburg-Eppendorf, Germany*
[2]*Molecular Parasitology Department, Bernard Nocht Institute for Tropical Medicine, Hamburg, Germany*

Purpose: The purpose of this study is to evaluate the labeling efficacy, migration behavior and in vivo distribution of the enteric parasite protozoan Entamoeba histolytica (E.h.) within the liver in MRI after injection in a mouse model. Non-invasive studies of migration and distribution of E.h. in the liver under different immunological constellations can help to understand the underlying mechanisms of amebic liver abscess formation.
Materials and Methods: In vitro magnetic labeling of E.h. was performed with commercially available superparamagnetic iron oxide nanoparticles (SPIO) with polyethylene glycol (PEG) coating (nano-screenMAG-PEG/P, Chemicell, Germany, hydrodynamic diameter 200 nm) by incubation for 48h in culture medium. Labeling efficiency and migration behavior of SPIO-E.h. was proven in MRI in vitro in culture medium in the static magnetic field of a preclinical 7T MRI system (ClinScan, Bruker) using T2w and T2*w dynamic susceptibility contrast MR sequences (DSC-MRI) for 88 hours (temporal resolution 4 min./image, effective voxel size 80x80x600 µm^3). Movement patterns were analyzed using ImageJ (NIH, USA). For in vivo experiments 10^5 SPIO-E.h. were injected in the left liver lobe of mice followed by serial respiration triggered T2*w and T2w MRI up to 3 days after injection. Furthermore ex vivo high resolution MRI was performed on removed liver specimens for in/ex-vivo comparison. MR images were matched with histology (PAS and Prussian Blue stains) as well as immunohistochemistry.
Results: Efficient magnetic labeling of E.h. could be performed by incubation with PEG-coated SPIO keeping the pathogenity and viability of E.h. In vitro dynamic MRI showed an undirected migration of single SPIO-E.h. in culture medium with pathogen movement in macroscopic dimensions with typical speeds of up to 4 mm/h. In vivo and ex vivo MRI of SPIO-E.h. showed strong E.h. presence at the site of amebic liver abscess formation and broad distribution within the left liver lobe, whereas no SPIO-E.h. could be detected in liver lobes different from lobe of injection. All MR findings were confirmed by histology.
Conclusion: Efficient magnetic labeling and non-invasive in vivo migration monitoring of pathogenic E.h. within the murine liver tissue is feasible in MRI.

Corresponding Author: H. Ittrich, ittrich@uke.de

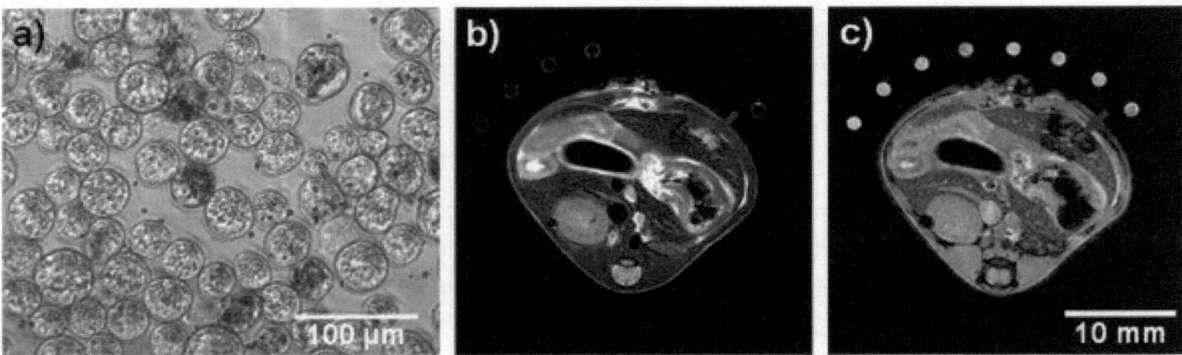

a) SPIO - labeled pathogen *Entamoeba histolytica* in light microscopy. b)+c) T2w fast spin echo image (b) and T2*w gradient echo image (c) of a transversal section of the mouse liver at day 3 post injection. An pronounced amebic liver abscess shows on b) while a broad distribution of SPIO - labeled *E.h.* in the left liver lobe can be observed on c).

Corresponding Author: H. Ittrich, ittrich@uke.de

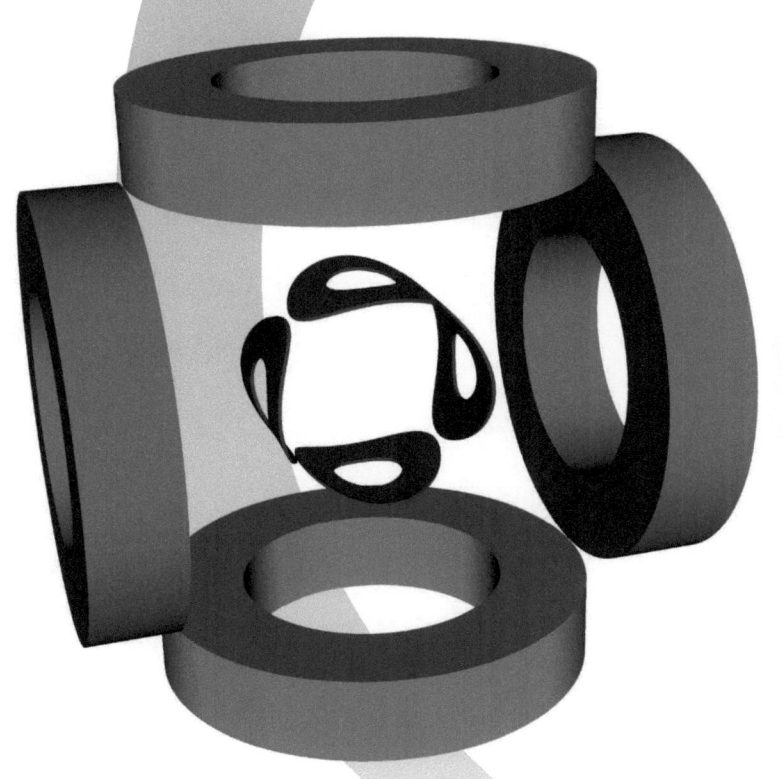

Magnetic Particle Imaging
IWMPI 2014

Infinite Science GmbH
MFC 1 | Technikzentrum Lübeck
BioMedTec Wissenschaftscampus
Maria-Goeppert-Straße 1
23562 Lübeck

www.iwmpi.org

info@iwmpi.org